Co

Fact Not Fiction

Volume II

Timeline and Chronology May 2020 - Aug 2020

Table of Contents

Dedication

For Shiv

Pandemic Chronology May 2020

1 May

- Australia has reported a total of about 6,700 cases and 93 deaths.
- Azerbaijan has reported a total of 1,804 cases and 24 deaths.
- China has reported 12 new cases (including six imported cases), bringing the total number of cases to over 84,000.
- France has reported 218 deaths, taking the total to 24,594. 25,887 remain in hospital and 3,878 in intensive care.
- Germany has reported 1,639 new cases, bringing the total to 160,758. The country has also reported 193 deaths, bringing the death toll to 6,481.
- Indonesia has reported 433 new cases, bringing the total number to 10,551. Indonesian health authorities have reported eight deaths, bringing the death toll to 800. Indonesia has reported 1,591 recoveries and has tested 76,500 people.
- Iran has reported 63 new deaths, bringing the death toll to 6,091. Iran has reported a total of 95,646 cases, with 2,899 in critical condition.
- Italy has reported 269 deaths, bringing the death toll to 28,236. Italy has announced 1,965 new cases, bringing the total to 207,428.
- Malaysia has reported 69 new cases (12 imported and 57 local transmissions), bringing the total number to 6,071. Malaysian authorities have also discharged 39 patients, bringing the number of recoveries to 4,210. Malaysia has

also reported a new death, bringing the country's death toll to 103.

- Mexico has reported 1,425 new cases, bringing the total to 19,224. Mexico has reported 127 new deaths, bringing the death toll to 1,859.
- The Netherlands has reported 475 new cases, bringing the total to 39,791. Dutch authorities have reported 98 new deaths, bringing the death toll to 4,893.
- New Zealand has reported three new cases, bringing the total to 1,479 (1,132 confirmed and 347 probable). NZ health authorities have also reported 11 new recoveries, bringing a total of 1,252.
- The Philippines has reported 284 new cases, bringing the total number to 8,772. The Philippines has reported 11 new deaths, bringing the death toll to 579.
- Qatar has reported 687 new cases, bringing the total number to 14,096. Qatar has also reported two new deaths, bringing the death toll to 12. A total of 1,436 people have recovered.
- Russia has reported 7,993 cases, bringing the total to 114,431. Russia has reported 96 deaths, bringing the death toll to 1,169.
- Singapore has reported 932 new cases, bringing the total to 17,101. Another death was later confirmed, bringing the total to 16.
- South Korea has reported nine new cases, bringing the total to 10,774, of which 9,072 have recovered.
- Spain has reported 281 deaths, bringing the death toll to 24,824. Spanish health authorities have also reported 1,781 new cases, bringing the total number of cases to 215,216.

- Thailand has reported six new cases, bringing the total number to 2,960. Thai authorities have reported no new deaths, with the death toll remaining at 54.
- Turkey has reported 84 deaths, bringing the death toll to 3,258. Turkey has reported 2,188 cases, bringing the total to 122,392.
- Ukraine has reported 455 new cases and 11 new deaths, bringing the total numbers to 10,861 and 272 respectively; a total of 1,413 patients have recovered.
- The United Kingdom has reported 279 deaths, bringing the death toll to 27,510. Health Secretary Matt Hancock announced that UK health authorities have conducted 122,347 tests, meeting its goal of testing 100,000 people.
- Matt Hancock confirms the government's target of providing (but not necessarily completing) 100,000 tests a day by the end of April has been met, with 122,347 provided over the previous 24 hours.
- Hancock announces that fertility clinics will be allowed to open again from 11 May.
- "Times Like These," a charity single by the Live Lounge Allstars released to raise funds for those affected by the pandemic, reaches number one in the UK Singles Chart.
- Facebook deletes the account of conspiracy theorist David Icke for posting misinformation about the coronavirus pandemic, including claims that it is being spread by the 5G network.
- In the United States, the estimated total death toll from the coronavirus is 63,000.

- Yemen has reported one new case in the Taiz governorate, bringing the total number to seven. Yemen has recorded a total of two deaths.
- According to Johns Hopkins University, there have been over 3.26 million cases, some 233,000 deaths, and more than one million recoveries.
- United States President Donald Trump noted about 63,000 have died in the US. He added that he would regard the virus' elimination and the reopening of the US economy as a victory.
- The Director of the National Institute of Allergy and Infectious Diseases, Dr. Anthony Fauci, has expressed optimism about Gilead Sciences' antiviral medication remdesivir after initial tests indicated it helped shorten recovery times. Later, the White House announced that Dr. Fauci will not be allowed to testify at a Congressional inquiry into the Trump Administration's handling of the coronavirus pandemic.
- Governor of New York Andrew Cuomo has announced that all schools and colleges in New York state will remain closed for the duration of the 2019–20 academic year.
- Texas and Ohio have embarked on a gradual relaxation of lockdown restrictions on Friday. Georgia has allowed all businesses to reopen.
- Several US airlines, including Southwest Airlines, Alaska Airlines, United Airlines, Delta Air Lines, the American Airlines Group, and Frontier Airlines, announced that all passengers will be required to wear face masks. Southwest Airlines has announced it will provide masks if patients forget to bring them.

- The stay-at-home orders in Marion County, Indiana, Davis County, Utah, and Summit County, Utah, are scheduled to end.
- South Africa has begun to loosen its lockdown restrictions, allowing some businesses and factories to resume operations. Restaurants will be allowed to provide takeaway services. Recreational activities such as walking, cycling, and running will be allowed for three hours a day. The South African Government has maintained a ban on the sales of cigarettes and alcohol.
- President of Zimbabwe Emmerson Mnangagwa has extended Zimbabwe's lockdown for two more weeks and announced a US$720 million stimulus for affected companies.
- Australian Prime Minister Scott Morrison announced that the Australian Government will make a decision by 8 May on whether to relax movement restrictions. Morrison also described Australia's relations with China as mutually beneficial in the face of tensions over Canberra, seeking an international inquiry into China's handling of the COVID-19 pandemic in Wuhan. Later, Morrison stated that he had no evidence to suggest that the coronavirus originated in a Wuhan laboratory.
- Chinese authorities announced that they will be reopening Beijing's Palace Museum on 1 May. Hubei provincial authorities announced that the province will lower its emergency response level from highest to second highest on 2 April.
- Japanese Prime Minister Shinzo Abe announced that the Japanese Government would decide by 4 May whether to

extend the country's state of emergency, which was set to expire on 6 May.

- The Philippines Government relaxed restrictions, placing areas with fewer cases under a more relaxed quarantine, allowing work, public transport, and businesses to resume operations at a reduced capacity.
- According to figures released by the South Korean Ministry of Trade, Industry, and Energy, South Korean exports declined by 24.3% in April 2020.
- World Health Organization spokesperson Tarik Jasarevic stated that WHO was seeking an invitation from China to participate in investigations into the animal origins of the coronavirus.
- Reactions and measures in South and Southeast Asia
- The Indian Government announces plans to make the contract tracing app Aarogya Setu compulsory for everything, including going to work and traveling on public transportation, raising concerns about privacy and surveillance from digital experts. The Indian Government also announced that they would extend the nationwide lockdown for two weeks after 4 May but would ease restrictions in lower-risk areas. Travel restrictions on air, rail, metro and inter-state movement by road remain suspended while schools, colleges, hotels, restaurants, shopping malls, cinemas, and places of worship remain closed.
- Indian authorities have also organised a special train transporting 1,200 migrant workers, who had been stranded as a result of lockdown measures, from Lingampally in the southern state of Telangana to Hatia in the eastern state of Jharkhand. During a video conference, several film

producers, directors, and actors opined that it would take two years for Bollywood to recover.

- Malaysian Prime Minister Muhyiddin Yassin announced that most businesses will be allowed to reopen from 4 May, with the exception of cinemas and bazaars since they involve large gatherings. Malaysian Transport Minister Dr. Wee Ka Siong confirmed that all public transportation services would resume on 4 May as part of the gradual relaxation of the country's movement control order. Human Rights Watch and the Asia Pacific Refugee Rights Network have reported that over 700 foreign migrant workers and refugees, including Rohingya, have been detained by Malaysian law enforcement authorities during the coronavirus pandemic.
- Azerbaijan extends lockdown measures until 31 May.
- French President Emmanuel Macron has announced that the end of the national lockdown on 11 May will mark the first step towards rebuilding the country's economy.
- In Germany, May Day protesters have defied a ban on social gatherings of more than 20 people by staging demonstrations in Berlin denouncing capitalism and calling for solidarity with refugees. Many protesters wore masks and stood at 1.5 meters apart.
- Hungarian Prime Minister Viktor Orbán has warned that Hungary needs to prepare for a potential second wave of the coronavirus between October and November during the autumn season. In addition, organisers for the 2020 Formula One World Championship in Hungary announced that the race will take place on 2 August without the spectators to comply with Hungarian social distancing rules.

- Irish Taoiseach Leo Varadkar has announced that people over the age of 70 will be permitted to go for short walks and drives from 5 May. Varadkar also announced that the Irish economy would open in five stages between 18 May and 10 August.
- Irish budget airliner Ryanair has announced that it plans to slash 3,000 inflight jobs as a result of the economic fallout of the coronavirus pandemic.
- Italian Prime Minister Giuseppe Conte has apologised for the Italian Government's delay in paying more than €$50 billion to assist struggling businesses and families.
- In Kazakhstan, Air Astana, SCAT, and Qazaq Air have resumed flight operations, but middle seats will be empty to ensure social distancing. Passengers will also be required to undergo temperature checks and present certificates confirming that they have tested negative for the coronavirus.
- Prime Minister of Slovakia Igor Matovic has lifted a quarantine placed on three Romani villages in April, which had been identified as clusters for the coronavirus.
- Spanish Economy and Business Minister Nadia Calviño has forecast that Spain's gross domestic product will contract by 9.2 percent in 2020.
- The Swiss Government is testing a contact tracing app on 100 Swiss Army soldiers prior to its planned launch on 11 May.
- The Turkish Government has evacuated 300 of its citizens overland from Baghdad and Iraq's southern provinces.
- In the United Kingdom, Heathrow Airport has reported a 12.7% drop in revenue to £593 million (US$754 million) in

the first quarter of 2020. Passenger numbers also declined by 97% as a result of the coronavirus pandemic. A report by the Institute of Fiscal Studies found that patients from the Bangladeshi, Pakistani, and Black ethnic communities had a higher mortality rate from the coronavirus than White Britons, reporting 2, 2.9, and 3.7 times the rate of white patients, respectively. Health Secretary Matt Hancock announced that UK health authorities have conducted 122,347 tests, meeting the British Government's goal of testing 100,000 people.

- The World Health Organization's (WHO) Director-General Tedros Adhanom has expressed "grace concerns" about the impact of the coronavirus on countries with "weaker health systems." The WHO emergencies chief Michael Ryan has stated that the coronavirus was of "natural origin," disputing US President Donald Trump's allegation that it had originated in a Chinese laboratory.
- South Africa has begun to loosen its lockdown restrictions, allowing some businesses and factories to resume operations. Restaurants will be allowed to provide takeaway services. Recreational activities such as walking, cycling, and running will be allowed for three hours a day. The South African Government has maintained a ban on the sales of cigarettes and alcohol.
- President of Zimbabwe Emmerson Mnangagwa has extended Zimbabwe's lockdown for two more weeks and announced a US$720 million stimulus for affected companies.
- Reactions and measures at the United Nations
- International experts on the COVID-19 Emergency Committee advised the World Health Organisation to work to

identify the animal origins of the virus causing the COVID-19 pandemic and its transmission to humans.

- The UN Secretary-General warned that the COVID-19 fatality rate for people over 80-years-old was five times the global average. He launched a new policy initiative tor challenges faced by the elderly as a result of "the biggest public health crisis to hit the world in a century."
- UNICEF warned of 'vaccine bottlenecks' and requested urgent help to distribute vaccines worldwide amid dramatic shortages because of COVID-19 restrictions.
- The International Civil Aviation Organization released figures warning of a potential reduction of 872 million international passengers to just over 1.3 billion in 2020.

2 May

- Africa Centres for Disease Control and Prevention (Africa CDC) has confirmed that Africa has recorded nearly 40,000 cases, nearly 1,700 deaths, and more than 13,000 recoveries. The coronavirus has occurred in 53 African countries.
- Australia has reported a total of nearly 6,800 cases and 93 deaths. Health authorities have identified a new cluster around a meat processing factory in the state of Victoria.
- Brazil has reported a total of 92,200 cases and 6,412 deaths.
- France has reported 166 deaths, bringing the death toll to 24,760.
- Germany has reported 954 cases, bringing the total to 161,703. Germany has also reported 94 deaths, bringing the death toll to 6,575.

- Italy has reported 474 deaths, bringing the death toll to 28,710. 1,539 remain in intensive care, while 79,914 have recovered.
- Malaysia has reported 105 new cases, bringing the total number to 6,176. In addition, 116 patients have been discharged, bringing the total number of recovered to 4,326. The death toll remains at 103.
- The Netherlands has reported 445 new cases, bringing the total to 40,236. The Dutch have reported 94 new deaths, bringing the death toll to 4,987.
- New Zealand has reported 6 new cases (2 confirmed and 4 probable), bringing the total to 1,485 (1,134 confirmed and 351 probable). NZ authorities have also reported 11 new recoveries, bringing the total to 1,263. NZ has also reported a new death, bringing the total to 20.
- The Philippines has reported 156 new cases, bringing the total to 8,928. The Philippines has reported 24 deaths, bringing the death toll to 603. 40 more people have recovered, bringing the total number of recovered to 1,124.
- Russia has reported 9,623 cases, bringing the total to 124,054. Russia has reported 57 deaths, bringing the death toll to 1,222. The Mayor of Moscow, Sergei Sobyanin, has also announced that 2 percent of Moscow's population (roughly 250,000 people) had tested positive for the coronavirus.
- Singapore has reported 447 new cases, bringing the total to 17,548. One death was later confirmed, bringing the total to 17. Another person was later confirmed to have COVID-19 after he died, which was caused by a heart attack.

- South Korea has reported six new cases, bringing the total to 10,780. The country has reported two new deaths, bringing the death toll to 250. 72 people have recovered, bringing the total to 9,123.
- Spain has reported 276 new deaths, bringing the death toll to 25,100. Spain has reported a total of 216,582 cases.
- Thailand has reported six new cases, bringing the total number to 2,966. The death toll remains at 54 while 2,732 have recovered and 180 remain in hospital.
- Turkey has reported a total of over 122,000 cases and 3,200 deaths.
- Ukraine has reported 550 new cases and 7 new deaths, bringing the total numbers to 11,411 and 279, respectively; a total of 1,498 patients have recovered.
- The United Kingdom has reported 621 deaths, bringing the total death toll to 28,131. England has reported 370 deaths (25 of whom had no underlying health conditions) in hospitals, bringing the death toll to 20,853.
- Robert Jenrick announces £76m of funding to help vulnerable people, including children, victims of domestic violence, and modern slavery, who may be "trapped in a nightmare" during the lockdown restrictions.
- YouTube becomes the latest social media platform to remove David Icke's official account.
- The United States has reported a total 65,645 deaths based on figures from Johns Hopkins University. The US also reported 34,000 cases, bringing the total number to more than 1.1 million. More than 164,000 people have recovered from the coronavirus, and 6.5 million tests have been conducted.

- Yemen has reported three new cases, bringing the total to ten. Yemen has reported a total of two deaths.
- There have been over 3.35 million cases, 239,000 deaths, and over 1.05 million recoveries globally.
- The Japan Sumo Association announced that it will reconsider rescheduling its grand summer tournament scheduled for 24 May if the Japanese Government decides to extend the nationwide lockdown, which was scheduled to end on 6 May.
- In the Philippines, Associate Justice of the Supreme Court Marvic Leonen confirmed that the Philippines Government released 9,731 prisoners, mainly those awaiting trial who could not afford bail, in an effort to ease the spread of the coronavirus in the country's overcrowded prison system.
- French Health Minister Olivier Véran has announced that the French Government will extend the country's health emergency by two months in order to combat the coronavirus.
- The Spanish Government has eased lockdown measures by allowing all Spaniards to for walks or play sports after 48 days of home confinement. Spanish Prime Minister Pedro Sánchez has announced that the government will make it compulsory to wear masks on public transportation. Madrid authorities have announced that they will distribute six million masks across the country from 4 May and another seven million to local authorities.
- The Turkish Ministry of Trade has lifted export limits on medical equipment and a requirement for public companies to obtain advance permission to export medical supplies and equipment overseas. Turkey has dispatched medical

supplies, including ventilators, to Somalia and the United States.

- The Indian Government has extended the country's coronavirus lockdown by two weeks.
- The United Nations in Malaysia's Head of Communications and Advocacy, Ahmad Hafiz Osman, called for migrants, refugees, asylum seekers, and stateless individuals in Malaysia to have access to health services and services without fear of repercussions.
- Health Minister Gan Kim Yong has announced that Singapore will lessen restrictions, including allowing some businesses to resume operations on 12 May and that some students will be allowed to return to school from 19 May.

3 May

- Afghanistan has reported a total of over 2,700 cases, 85 deaths and conducted nearly 12,000 tests. Afghan health authorities have also confirmed that 500 random tests in the capital Kabul identified 150 positive tests.
- Armenia has reported a total of 2,386 cases and 35 deaths.
- Brazil has reported 4,588 new cases, bringing the total to 101,147. Brazil has reported 275 deaths, bringing the death toll to 7,025.
- Canada has reported 160 new deaths, bringing the death toll to 3,606. Canada has reported 1,576 new cases, bringing the total to 57,148.
- China has reported two new cases and 12 new asymptomatic cases, bringing the total to 82,877. The death toll remains at 4,633.

- France has reported 135 new deaths, bringing the death toll to 24,895. 25,815 remain in hospital and 3,819 in intensive care, down from 25,827 and 3,827, respectively.
- India has reported 2,644 new cases, bringing the total to over 39,000. India has reported 83 new deaths, bringing the death toll to 1,301.
- Indonesia has reported 349 new cases, bringing the total to 11,912. Indonesia has reported 18 deaths, bringing the death toll to 845.
- Iran has reported 47 new deaths, bringing the death toll to 6,203. Iran has reported a total of 97,424 cases.
- Israel has reported a total of 16,194 cases and 230 deaths.
- Italy has reported 174 deaths, bringing the death toll to 28,884. Italy has reported 1,389 cases, bringing the total to 210,717.
- Malaysia has reported 122 new cases, bringing the total number to 6,297. Malaysian health authorities have also reported two new deaths, bringing the death toll to 105.
- The Netherlands has reported 335 new cases, bringing the total to 40,471. The Dutch have reported 69 new deaths, bringing the total to 5,056.
- New Zealand has reported two new cases, bringing the total to 1,487 (1,136 confirmed and 351 probable). NZ health authorities have also reported three new recoveries, bringing the total to 1,266.
- The Philippines has reported a total of 9,223 cases and 607 deaths.
- Qatar has reported 679 cases, bringing the total to 15,551. The country has reported a total of 12 deaths.
- Russia has reported 10,633 new cases.

- Singapore has reported 657 new cases, bringing the total to 18,205. In addition, Singapore's Ministry of Health attributed the fluctuation of cases in recent days to a case backlog in a laboratory, with steps to fix that in progress. One death was later confirmed, bringing the total to 18.
- South Korea has reported 13 new cases, 10 of which have been imported.
- Thailand has reported three new cases, bringing the total to 2,966. The country has reported a total of 54 deaths.
- Turkey has reported 61 deaths, bringing the death toll to 3,397. Turkey has reported 1,670 new cases, bringing the total to 120,045. A total of 63,151 have recovered.
- Ukraine has reported 502 new cases and 9 new deaths, bringing the total numbers to 11,913 and 288, respectively; a total of 1,547 patients have recovered.
- The United Kingdom has reported 315 deaths, bringing the death toll to 28,446, including hospitals, care homes, and community figures.
- In an interview with the Sun on Sunday, Boris Johnson speaks about how contingency plans were made for the event of his death while he was in intensive care.
- An NHS contact tracing app designed to track and prevent the spread of COVID-19 will be trialed on the Isle of Wight during the forthcoming week.
- In the United States, Virginia has reported its first death due to the virus, bringing the total deaths in the United States to 65,646.
- Vietnam has reported its first new case in nine days, bringing the total to 271. More than 30,500 people have been quarantined, and 261,000 have been tested.

- Brazilian authorities have managed to restore order following an uprising at Puraquequara prison in Manaus, where seven guards were taken hostage by prisoners protesting poor living conditions. Ten guards and five prisoners suffered non-critical injuries during the uprising.
- United States President Donald Trump has expressed confidence that there will be a coronavirus vaccine by the end of 2020 during a media interview. He also expressed hope that schools and universities will reopen in September.
- United States Secretary of State Mike Pompeo has claimed that there is "enormous evidence" that COVID-19 originated in a laboratory in Wuhan.
- Democratic US Speaker of the House of Representatives Nancy Pelosi and Republican Senate Majority Leader Mitch McConnell have declined an offer for quick COVID-19 tests from the Trump Administration, stating that these resources are needed at the frontline.
- New York Governor Andrew Cuomo has thanked Qatar for sending critical supplies and aid to New York State.
- In Oregon, hundreds have staged protests in the state capital Salem protesting against lockdown measures.
- Swiss multinational health company Hoffman-La Roche has received approval from the US Food and Drug Administration to conduct its antibody test Elecsys Anti-SARS-CoV-2 on people. This antibody test will test whether people have been infected with the coronavirus and assess their immune system's response to the coronavirus.
- The Philippines banned incoming flights for one week. 20,000 repatriated Filipinos underwent mandatory quarantine.

- Thailand eased restrictions on restaurants, hair salons, and outdoor markets as long as they adhere to social distancing rules and conduct temperature tests.
- South Korean Prime Minister Chung Sye-Kyun announced the easing of social distancing restrictions, allowing businesses to reopen and allow public gatherings to take place provided they followed disinfection guidelines.
- Armenian Deputy Prime Minister Tigran Avinyan has allowed shops, restaurants, and bars to resume as part of the relaxation of its lockdown policies in order to ease the economic fallout of the coronavirus pandemic.
- In Austria, Vienna Airport announced that it will offer onsite coronavirus testing from Monday in order to minimise the risk of inbound passengers being quarantined. The test will cost €190 (US$209) and would be available in two to three hours.
- Hungarian budget airline Wizz Air has announced that it will resume flights from European cities to Abu Dhabi from June 2020.
- Israel has allowed first, second, and third-grade students as well as students in the last two grades of high school to return to classes, which had been shut down in mid-March in order to contain the spread of the coronavirus.
- United Kingdom Prime Minister Boris Johnson has acknowledged during a media interview that the British Government had made contingency plans in the event of his death from the coronavirus. Minister for the Cabinet Office Michael Gove announced that the British Government will also test a new coronavirus tracing programme in the Isle of Wight.

- Iranian President Hassan Rouhani has announced that mosques in 312 Iranian counties will reopen but would have to comply with social distancing rules.
- The Jordanian Government has lifted all restrictions on economic activity, including social distancing and health measures, in order to jump-start the country's economy.
- The Palestinian stock exchange has resumed trading after 40 days of inactivity as part of the Palestinian Authority's efforts to relax lockdown restrictions. Chief Executive Ahmad Aweidah has announced that investors will be allowed to trade remotely in line with health regulations.
- In the United Arab Emirates, three shopping centres in Abu Dhabi have reopened after adopting safety measures, including social distancing and installing thermal inspection devices.
- In Yemen, the Houthi Health Minister Taha Al-Mutawakel has appealed for the United Nations to send them more test kits due to the country's acute economic situation resulting from the Yemeni Civil War and sanctions.

4 May

- Bangladesh has reported 688 new cases, bringing the total to 10,143. The country has reported a total of 182 deaths.
- Brazil has reported 4,075 new cases, bringing the total to 105,222. Brazil has reported 263 deaths, bringing the death toll to 7,288.
- Chile has reported 980 new cases, bringing the total to 20,643. The country also reported 10 new deaths, bringing the total to 270.

- China has reported three new cases, bringing the total to 82,880. China has also reported 13 new asymptomatic cases.
- Germany has reported 679 new cases, bringing the total to 163,175. Germany has reported 43 deaths, bringing the death toll to 6,692.
- Indonesia has reported 395 new cases, bringing the total to 11,587. Indonesian health ministry official Achmad Yurianto has also confirmed 19 new deaths, bringing the total to 864. A total of 1,954 have recovered.
- Iran has reported 74 new deaths, bringing the death toll to 6,277. Iran has reported a total of 98,647 cases.
- Israel has reported 38 new cases, bringing the total number to 16,246. Three people have died, bringing the death toll to 233. A total of 10,064 people have recovered, and 6,436 people have been tested.
- Italy has reported 195 new deaths, bringing the death toll to 29,079. Italy reported 1,221 new cases, bringing the total to 211,938. 99,980 remain infected, with 1,479 in intensive care. 82,879 have recovered, and 1.48 million have been tested for COVID-19.
- Malaysia has reported 55 new cases, bringing the total to 6,353. 71 people have been discharged, bringing the number of recovered to 4,484. Malaysia has reported no new deaths, with the death toll remaining at 105.
- The Netherlands has reported 199 new cases, bringing the total to 40,770. Dutch authorities reported 26 new deaths, bringing the death toll to 5,082.
- New Zealand has reported no new cases, but one probable case was reclassified as confirmed, keeping the total at

1,487 (1,137 confirmed and 350 probable). In addition, NZ health authorities have confirmed ten new recoveries, bringing the total to 1,276.

- The Philippines has reported 16 new deaths, bringing the death toll to 623. The Philippines has also reported 262 new cases, bringing the total to 9,485.
- Russia has reported 10,581 new cases.
- Singapore has reported 573 new cases, bringing the total to 18,778.
- South Korea has reported eight new cases, bringing the total to 10,801.
- Turkey has reported 65 deaths, bringing the death toll to 3,461. Turkish authorities have reported 1,614 new cases, bringing the total to 127,659. A total of 68,166 people have recovered. Turkey has conducted 35,771 new tests, bringing the total number of tests to 1.170 million.
- Ukraine has reported 418 new cases and 15 new deaths, bringing the total numbers to 12,331 and 303 respectively; a total of 1,619 patients have recovered.
- The United Kingdom has reported 288 deaths, bringing the death toll to 28,734.
- Yemen has reported two new cases, bringing the total to 12. The country has a total of two deaths.
- Apple and Google approve a test version of the NHS tracing app.
- Businessman Simon Dolan announces that he will seek a court injunction to lift the lockdown in Britain.
- According to an Al Jazeera report, the Trump Administration is seeking to accelerate efforts to reduce production and

supply chain dependence on China and is considering new tariffs.

- The White House has rebuffed a New York Times report forecasting that the United States could experience 3,000 deaths per day by June 2020 as the United States economy reopens. The New York Times report had cited an internal White House document based on government modeling compiled by the Federal Emergency Management Agency, forecasting 200,000 cases per day by late May. The White House claimed that the document had not been presented to the Coronavirus Task Force or undergone inter-agency vetting.
- Director of the Office of Trade and Manufacturing Policy Peter Navarro confirmed that the Trump Administration would be introducing an executive order requiring federal agencies to purchase US-made medical products.
- New York Governor Andrew Cuomo announced that the state will be reopening its economy in stages, beginning with manufacturing and construction, without announcing dates.
- Secretary-General of the United Nations António Guterres has called for any treatment for the coronavirus to be made available to anyone.
- The International Monetary Fund has disbursed Cameroon US$226 million to meet the urgent balance of payment needs caused by the COVID-19 pandemic.
- In South Africa, Dondo Mogajane, the Director-General of the National Treasury, has warned that the South African economy could contract by 12% and that one-third of the workforce could be affected by the coronavirus as a result of the economic fallout of the COVID-19 pandemic.

- Zimbabwean Finance and Economic Development Minister Mthuli Ncube have appealed for the International Monetary Fund to clear its debt arrears in order to access foreign funding for COVID-19 relief efforts.
- Several Brazilian indigenous leaders, including Joenia Wapichana, have appealed to World Health Organization Director-General Tedros Adhanom for help in establishing an emergency fund to provide personal protective equipment to health workers in tribal reservations and villages.
- United States President Donald Trump has announced that the US Government will release a report into the origins of the coronavirus in the near future without specifying a date. Later, Trump announced that the White House Coronavirus Task Force would be winding down as the country shifted to reopening the US economy.
- White House Coronavirus Task Force adviser Dr. Anthony Fauci stated there was no scientific evidence that the coronavirus originated in a Chinese laboratory during an interview with National Geographic.
- Former Director of the Biomedical Advanced Research and Development Authority Dr. Rick Bright has filed a whistleblower complaint claiming that the Trump Administration had dismissed him after ignoring his initial warnings about the COVID-19 pandemic and his opposition to the use of the anti-malaria drug hydroxychloroquine to treat the coronavirus.
- Researchers at the University of Washington's Institute for Health Metrics and Evaluation (IHME) have released a new coronavirus mortality model predicting that 135,000 Americans will die from COVID-19 by early August 2020 as

a result of the relaxation of social distancing measures. An earlier model released on 29 April had predicted 72,400 deaths.

- The US-based public relations company Edelman released its 2020 Edelman Trust Barometer, showing that 64% of respondents were aware of the rich-poor divide as a result of the COVID-19 pandemic; 67% felt that the less educated, poor, and less-resourced were disproportionately affected by the pandemic; 67% were worried about "biased and inaccurate" information being spread about the coronavirus; and that 67% believed that the government should prioritize saving lives over the economy. Only 33% of respondents globally thought it was more important to save jobs and the economy. Edelman surveyed more than 13,200 respondents in Canada, China, France, Germany, India, Japan, Mexico, Saudi Arabia, South Korea, the United Kingdom, and the United States between April 15 and April 23.
- Canada and the US are likely to extend a ban on non-essential travel across the border until June 21, as revealed to Reuters by top Canadian and American officials. Canada is allegedly pushing for the measures to be extended for another month, with the restrictions due to end on May 21.
- The President of the New York Stock Exchange, Stacey Cunningham, announced that the trading floor will partially open on May 26.
- The US Secretary of State Mike Pompeo has condemned attempts by "cyber actors and non-traditional collectors affiliated with China" to steal American data linked to the coronavirus. The Chinese embassy in Washington described the accusation as "lies." Donald Trump said in an interview

with Fox Business Network that he was "very disappointed in China; they should never have let this happen."

- The US Labor Department reports that nearly three million Americans applied for unemployment benefits the previous week. Roughly 36 million Americans filed for unemployment benefits in the first two months of the pandemic
- The Supreme Court of the US state of Wisconsin had repealed the stay-at-home order issued by Governor Tony Evers, ruling that his administration surpassed its authoritative powers when the order was extended for an additional month without consulting legislators. This ruling effectively reopened the state, lifting limits on social gatherings, allowing travel, and allowing businesses and restaurants to reopen. President Donald Trump applauded the news.
- In Australia, New South Wales began opening schools. New South Wales Premier Gladys Berejiklian confirmed that a seven-year-old boy had tested positive for COVID-19, and the school was closed.
- The Associated Press reported that a United States Department of Homeland Security report dated 1 May states that intelligence officials believed that China covered up the extent of the COVID-19 outbreak to allow time for them to stock up on supplies.
- Chinese state broadcaster China Central Television issued a statement accusing United States Secretary of State Mike Pompeo of "wantonly spewing poison and spreading lies" about the origins of the COVID-19 pandemic in response to Pompeo's statement claiming that the coronavirus had originated in a laboratory in Wuhan.

- Japanese Economic Minister Yasutoshi Nishimura announced the extension of the state of emergency, due to expiring on 6 May, until 31 May.
- New Zealand Prime Minister Jacinda Ardern met with Australian Prime Minister Scott Morrison via video conference. Topics include the possible creation of an Australian-New Zealand travel bubble.
- The South Korean Education Minister Yoo Eun-hae announced that South Korea will reopen schools in stages from 13 May. She also indicated that schools might switch to online learning if a student contracts COVID-19.
- FINA (the International Swimming Federation) postponed the 2021 World Aquatics Championships, scheduled for Fukuoka, Japan, in May 2021 to 13–29 May 2022.
- The Indian Government has indicated that it will begin to ease lockdown restrictions. The Indian government has colour-coded states and cities into red, orange, and green zones based on the number of cases. Each type of zone has different levels of restrictions. All travel is forbidden, and schools, shopping malls, hotels, and public spaces remain closed.
- The Malaysian federal government has allowed businesses, including restaurants, to reopen. Due to a spike of cases over the weekends, some state governments have indicated that they will not ease restrictions.
- The Bureau International des Expositions (BIE) has voted to delay Expo 2020 in Dubai to between 1 October 2021 and 31 March 2022.

- Syrian President Bashar Al-Assad has warned that Syria faces a "real catastrophe" if the number of COVID-19 cases rises and overwhelms health services.
- The World Health Organization welcomed a 7.4 billion Euro pledge by world leaders for COVID-19 treatments. At the same time, the UN Secretary-General warned that five times that amount would be required, urging the "most massive public health effort in history."
- At a UNESCO-led event to mark World Press Freedom Day, the UN Secretary-General noted that journalists are key to countering the "dangerous outbreak of misinformation" accompanying the COVID-19 pandemic, including harmful health advice, hate speech, wild conspiracy theories, and "blatant lies."
- The European Commission has approved €7 billion in French state aid to help beleaguered national carrier Air France cushion the economic fallout of the coronavirus pandemic. Later that day, President of the European Commission Ursula von der Leyen announced that the European Union was pledging €1 billion (US$1.09) to finance global research into treatment and vaccines for COVID-19 during an online pledging event. In total, world leaders have pledged €7.4 billion into supporting research into researching vaccines, diagnostics, and treatment of COVID-19.
- The Finnish Government announced that they will be lifting COVID-19 restrictions, allowing restaurants, libraries, sports facilities, and public services to resume from 1 June. Public gatherings of 50 people will also be allowed from 1 June. Essential travel to Schengen Area countries will be allowed from 14 May.

- French President Emmanuel Macron and German Chancellor Angela Merkel have announced that their governments will contribute €500 million and €525 million respectively to global fundraising initiatives to finance research into vaccines and treatment for the coronavirus.
- The German Health Minister Jens Spahn has warned that it could take years to develop a vaccine for COVID-19 in response to remarks by President Trump that they could have a vaccine by late 2020. ,e. The German government allowed museums, hairdressers, churches, and car factories to reopen that day.
- Israeli Prime Minister Benjamin Netanyahu has announced that Israel will be easing several lockdown restrictions, including allowing visits to immediate family members, allowing public gatherings of up to 20 people in open areas (to be expanded to 50 people on 17 May), and allowing weddings and funerals of up to 50 people in open areas. Malls and outdoor markets will be allowed to reopen on 7 May. Netanyahu also announced that the process for small businesses and the self-employed will be eased. Kindergartens will reopen on 10 May, and all schools are expected to reopen by the end of May. Universities and colleges are set to reopen on 14 June. Restrictions on recreational activities will also be used.
- In Italy, 4.4 million people have returned to work after the Italian Government eased lockdown restrictions after seven weeks of a nationwide lockdown.
- Romanian President Klaus Iohannis has announced that Romania will not extend the state of emergency beyond 15 May but will a "state of alert" allowing some moderate easing

of restrictions, including lifting travel restrictions for groups of three or less. Public gatherings remain banned.

- In Switzerland, environmentalists have delivered a 22,000 petition to the Federal Assembly demanding that the Swiss Government pass a US$64 billion aid package encouraging "green recovery" and demanding that state support be tied to reducing carbon emissions.
- Turkish President Recep Tayyip Erdoğan announced that Turkey will be relaxing lockdown restrictions in May, June, and July. He announced that young people and senior citizens will be allowed to spend four hours outside a day from the weekend onwards. Travel restrictions were lifted in some cities. Some shops and services will be allowed to reopen on May 11, while universities will reopen on 15 June. However, Erdoğan warned that the Turkish Government would impose harsher measures if citizens did not abide by the normalisation plan.
- The Ukrainian Government has extended the nationwide lockdown until 22 May. Still, it has eased health restrictions, including reopening parks, recreational areas, shops specialising in household goods and textiles, and eateries for takeaways.
- In the United Kingdom, a spokesperson for British Prime Minister Boris Johnson stated that research was needed regarding the origin and spread of COVID-19 in order to prepare for future pandemics. Deputy Chief Medical Officer Jonathan Van-Tam issued a statement at a press conference that the UK would only ease lockdown restrictions once the number of cases had started to decline. Van-Tam also confirmed that most coronavirus patients

developed antibodies against COVID-19, but results were still too early to indicate whether they provided immunity.

- World Health Organization Director-General Tedros Adhanom called for the world to work together to defeat COVID-19, praising recent pledges of US$8 billion by world leaders to combat the pandemic.
- The International Monetary Fund has disbursed Cameroon US$226 million to meet the urgent balance of payment needs caused by the COVID-19 pandemic.
- In South Africa, Dondo Mogajane, the Director-General of the National Treasury, has warned that the South African economy could contract by 12% and that one-third of the workforce could be affected by the coronavirus as a result of the economic fallout of the COVID-19 pandemic.
- Zimbabwean Finance and Economic Development Minister Mthuli Ncube has appealed for the International Monetary Fund to clear its debt arrears in order to access foreign funding for COVID-19 relief efforts.

5 May

- Brazil has reported 6,935 new cases, bringing the total to 114,715. Health authorities have also reported 600 new deaths, bringing the total to 7,921.
- China has reported one new case and 15 asymptomatic cases.
- France has reported 330 deaths, bringing the death toll to 25,531. 25,755 people remain in hospital, with 3,430 in intensive care, down from 25,548 and 3,696, respectively.

- Germany has reported 685 new cases, bringing the total to 139,860. Germany has also reported 139 deaths, bringing the total to 6,831.
- Indonesia has reported 484 cases, bringing the total to 12,071.
- Iran has reported 1,323 new cases, bringing the total to 99,970. Iranian health authorities have also reported 63 deaths, bringing the death toll to 6,340.
- Italy has reported 236 new deaths, bringing the death toll to 29,315. Italy has reported 1,075 new cases, bringing the total to 213,013.
- Madagascar has reported a total of 149 cases and no deaths.
- Malaysia has reported 30 new cases, bringing the total to 6,883. 83 patients have been discharged, bringing the total number of recoveries to 4,567. Malaysia has reported one new death, bringing the death toll to 106.
- New Zealand has reported no new cases, and one previous probable case was rescinded, bringing the total down to 1,486 (1,137 confirmed and 349 probable). 26 new recoveries have been reported, bringing the total to 1,302.
- Peru has reported a total of 51,189 cases and 1,444 deaths.
- The Philippines has reported 14 new deaths, bringing the death toll to 637. Health authorities have also reported 199 new cases, bringing the total number to 9,684. 93 patients have recovered, bringing the total to 1,408.
- Russia has reported 10,102 new cases, bringing the total to 155,370. Russia has also reported 95 deaths, bringing the death toll to 1,451.

- Singapore has reported 632 new cases, bringing the total to 19,410. In addition, a patient who had COVID-19 died from a heart attack.
- Spain has reported 185 deaths, bringing the death toll to 25,428. The country has reported a total of 219,329 cases.
- Sudan has reported four new deaths, bringing the death toll to 45. Sudanese authorities have reported 100 new cases, bringing the total to 778. 70 people have recovered from the coronavirus.
- Thailand has reported one new case, bringing the total number to 2,988. Thailand has reported no new deaths, with the death toll remaining at 54. 2,747 have recovered, while 84 are still being treated in hospitals.
- Turkey has reported 59 deaths, bringing the death toll to 3,250. Turkey has also reported 1,832 new cases, bringing the total to 129,491.
- Ukraine has reported 366 new cases and 13 new deaths, bringing the total numbers to 12,697 and 316 respectively; a total of 1,875 patients have recovered.
- The United Kingdom has reported over 30,000 deaths, including 29,648 deaths in England and Wales.
- The number of recorded deaths rises by 693 to 29,427, giving the UK the highest number of COVID-19 related deaths in Europe.
- Figures from the Office for National Statistics for the week ending 24 April show 21,997 deaths from all causes registered in England and Wales; this is a decrease of 354 from the previous week but still nearly twice the five-year average for the time of year. Deaths per week in hospitals are falling while those in care homes continue to increase,

and for the year to 24 April, 5,890 deaths in care homes involved COVID-19.

- Trials of the NHS contact-tracing app start on the Isle of Wight, with the app being made available to healthcare and council workers.
- NHS Nightingale Hospital North East, a temporary critical care hospital built near Sunderland for COVID-19 patients, is officially opened by Health Secretary Matt Hancock. The virtual ceremony features TV celebrities Ant and Dec, football pundit Alan Shearer and cricketer Ben Stokes.
- Figures from the Society of Motor Manufacturers and Traders (SMMT) indicate that just 4,321 new cars were registered in April, the lowest monthly number since 1946 and a 97% fall in sales from April 2019; 70% of new cars for the month were company fleet vehicles.
- Airline operator Virgin Atlantic announces it has shed more than 3,000 jobs and ended operations at Gatwick Airport as a result of the COVID-19 outbreak, as well as withdrawing all their Boeing 747 fleet.
- Sir Patrick Vallance tells the House of Commons Health Select Committee earlier testing for COVID-19 would have been "beneficial" but would not have prevented the spread of the virus.
- Professor Neil Ferguson, whose advice led the government to implement the lockdown restrictions, resigned from the Scientific Advisory Group for Emergencies after the Daily Telegraph reports a woman named his "married lover" visited his home during the restrictions.
- The United States has reported a total of 70,115 deaths, 1,192,119 cases, and 187,000 recoveries. The hardest-hit

states are New York (27,073 deaths and over 321,000 cases) and New Jersey (8,244 deaths and over 130,600 cases).

- Yemen has reported nine new cases, bringing the total to 21 and three deaths. The Houthi–controlled government in Sanaa has reported its first case, a Somali man, and death.
- According to figures released by Johns Hopkins University, the number of global coronavirus cases has exceeded 3.5 million, 251,718 have died, and 1.2 million have recovered.
- The World Health Organization and the US Centers for Disease Control have urged people not to try untested remedies in response to Madagascan President Andry Rajoelina promoting an untested herbal remedy called COVID-Organicswas produced from Artemesia and other indigenous herbs by the Malagasy Institute of Applied Research.
- The World Health Organization and the US Centers for Disease Control have urged people not to try untested remedies in response to Madagascan President Andry Rajoelina promoting an untested herbal remedy called COVID-Organics, which was produced from Artemesia and other indigenous herbs by the Malagasy Institute of Applied Research.
- The Indian Government has announced that it will repatriate 190,000 Indian nationals over the next several weeks, including the Middle East. In the first week, the Indian Government intends to bring back 14,800 nationals from 12 countries, including the United States, Britain, the United Arab Emirates, Saudi Arabia, Qatar, Kuwait, Bangladesh, the Philippines, Singapore, and Malaysia. The Indian Navy

has also diverted three ships to bring back 1,000 Indian nationals from the Maldives and the Middle East.

- The Australian and New Zealand Prime Ministers Scott Morrison and Jacinda Ardern, along with several Australian state and territorial leaders, pledged to work together to develop a trans-Tasman COVID-safe travel zone that would allow residents from both countries to travel freely without travel restrictions. Ardern, , has ruled out including the Pacific Islands within this travel bubble, citing the danger of COVID-19 spreading to unaffected Pacific states. During a media conference, Morrison stated that the coronavirus most likely originated in a wet wildlife market in Wuhan instead of a laboratory while supporting calls for an inquiry into the origins of the COVID-19 pandemic in Wuhan.
- The South Korean government allowed professional sporting bodies, including the Korea Baseball Organization, to resume professional sports in empty stadiums.
- The Afghan Government has distributed free bread to hundreds of thousands of Afghans due to the disruption of food supplies and inflation caused by the COVID-19 pandemic. As part of the project's first phase, over 250,000 families in Kabul have received ten flat pieces of Naan bread a day.
- The Jordanian Government has announced that it will maintain night curfews, which were imposed on 21 March.
- The Palestinian Authority has extended a state of emergency in the West Bank by one month. Under the state of emergency, Palestinians have been confined to their homes except for essential travel. UNRWA (the United Nations Relief and Works Agency for Palestine Refugees in the Near East) has warned that the agency only has enough

cash to continue covering operating expenditures, including paying 30,000 healthcare workers until the end of May 2020 due to American funding cuts.

- In the United Arab Emirates, the vehicle for hire company Careem, a subsidiary of Uber, has cut 31 percent of its workforce (536 employees) as a result of the economic fallout of the COVID-19 pandemic.
- The International Telecommunications Union outlined the implications of the pandemic, warning that it was essential to bridge the digital divide for the 3.6 billion off-line people while internet traffic had tripled.
- As COVID-19 restrictions worsened people's vulnerability, the World Food Programme warned well over 40 million people across West Africa faced desperate food shortages.
- The UN Special Rapporteur on the Contemporary Forms of Slavery warned that the COVID-19 pandemic was worsening global slavery.
- European Commissioner for Internal Market Thierry Breton has denied that the European Union has been "naive" in its dealings with China during a France Info radio interview.
- French Secretary of State for the Digital Economy Cédric O has announced that the French Government plans to launch its "StopCOVID" contact tracing app by 2 June. French President Emmanuel Macron has warned that travel within the European Union and abroad will be limited during the summer of 2020 in order to minimise the risk of the resurgence of COVID-19.
- Several German states have eased lockdown requirements despite German Chancellor Angela Merkel's pleas for "prudence" in efforts to contain the COVID-19 pandemic.

- Hungarian budget airliner Wizz Air reported a 98 decline in passenger numbers in April as a result of the COVID-19 pandemic, with the airline carrying 78,389 passengers that month.
- An Israeli Knesset panel has allowed the country's domestic intelligence agency Shin Bet to continue using mobile phone data to track the movements of coronavirus patients until 26 May.
- In the Netherlands, the Mayor of the Hague ordered police to disperse a 200-strong protest against the country's lockdown measures, detaining dozens of protesters. Dutch scientists have also identified an antibody capable of resisting the coronavirus during lab tests.
- Turkish Industry and Technology Minister Mustafa Varank announced that all major Turkish automotive factories can resume operations from 11 May.
- The United Kingdom's National Cyber Security Centre (NCSC) and the United States' Cybersecurity and Infrastructure Security Agency (CISA) issued a joint statement stating that government-backed hackers had been targeting pharmaceutical companies, research organisations, and local governments in order to steal information about efforts to combat the COVID-19 pandemic. Iran, China, and Russia have denied any role in these attacks and have claimed to be the victims of similar cyber attacks. British carrier Virgin Atlantic has announced that it will slash over 3,000 jobs as a result of the economic fallout of the coronavirus pandemic.
- World Health Organization spokesperson Christian Lindmeier stated that there may be more earlier reports of

the coronavirus after a French hospital discovered it had treated a man with COVID-19 on 27 December after retesting pneumonia patients samples, nearly a month before French health authorities confirmed the country's first case.

- Tajikistan's Health Minister Nasim Olimzoda resigns over allegations that the Tajik Government had downplayed the seriousness of the coronavirus pandemic.
- The World Health Organization and the US Centers for Disease Control have urged people not to try untested remedies in response to Madagascan President Andry Rajoelina promoting an untested herbal remedy called COVID-Organics, which was produced from Artemesia and other indigenous herbs by the Malagasy Institute of Applied Research.

6 May

- Canada has reported a total of 4,111 deaths and 62,458 cases.
- China has reported two new cases and 20 new asymptomatic cases.
- In Ecuador, the Secoya tribe (also known as the Siekopai) has reported 15 cases among their population of 744.
- France has reported 4,183 new cases. French authorities have also reported 278 new deaths (181 in hospitals and 97 in nursing homes), bringing the death toll to 16,237. 24,983 remain in hospital, with 3,147 in intensive care.
- Germany has reported 947 cases, bringing the total to 164,807. 165 have died, bringing the death toll to 6,996.

- Iran has reported 1,680 new cases, bringing the total number beyond the 100,000 mark.
- Italy has reported 369 deaths, bringing the death toll to 29,684. Italy has reported 1,444 cases, bringing the total to 214,457. 91,528 remained infected, with 1,333 in intensive care. 1.550 million people have been tested.
- Malaysia has reported 45 new cases, bringing the total to 6,248. Malaysia has discharged 135 patients, bringing the number of recoveries to 4,702. Malaysia has also reported one new death, bringing the death toll to 107.
- New Zealand has reported two new cases (1 confirmed and 1 probable), bringing the total to 1,488 (1,138 confirmed and 350 probable). NZ health authorities have reported 14 new recoveries, bringing the total to 1,316. New Zealand has reported one new death, bringing the death toll to 21.
- The Philippines has reported 320 new cases, bringing the total to 10,004. The Philippines has reported 21 new deaths, bringing the death toll to 658.
- Qatar has reported 830 cases, bringing the total to 15,890. The total number of recoveries is 2,070.
- Russia has reported 10,559 cases, bringing the total to 165,929. Russia has reported 86 deaths, bringing the death toll to 1,537.
- Singapore has reported 788 new cases, bringing the total to 20,198. Two deaths have been confirmed, bringing the death toll to 20.
- Slovakia has reported a total of 1,429 cases and 25 deaths, with recoveries being about half the total number of cases.
- South Ossetia has reported its first three cases.

- Spain has reported 244 deaths, bringing the death toll to 25,857. Spain has reported 996 new cases, bringing the total to 220,325.
- Turkey has reported 64 new deaths, bringing the death toll to 3,584. Turkey has reported 2,253 new cases, bringing the total to 131,744. A total of 78,202 have recovered.
- At his first Prime Minister's Questions since returning to work, Boris Johnson says he "bitterly regrets" the crisis in care homes and is "working very hard" to tackle it. Johnson also pledges to reach a target of 200,000 daily UK coronavirus tests by the end of May.
- A further 649 deaths take the number of recorded deaths over 30,000 to 30,076.
- John Holland-Kaye, the CEO of Heathrow Airport, tells the Transport Select Committee that the airport is trialling large-scale temperature checks at departure gates.
- Ukraine has reported 487 new cases and 11 new deaths, bringing the total numbers to 13,184 and 327, respectively; a total of 2,097 patients have recovered.
- The International Council of Nurses has reported that 90,000 nurses have been affected, with 260 killed.
- Yemen has reported three deaths and 25 cases.
- US President Donald Trump has denied earlier reports that the White House Coronavirus Task Force would be disbanded, stating that its work would continue "indefinitely." He confirmed that Dr. Anthony Fauci and Task Force coordinator Deborah Birx will continue to serve on the Task Force.

- United States Secretary of Agriculture Sonny Perdue has also announced that US meat processing plants would be fully operational within ten days.
- United States Secretary of State Mike Pompeo issued a statement accusing China of covering up the initial outbreak in Wuhan and causing hundreds of thousands of deaths and a global economic malaise.
- New York Governor Andrew Cuomo has criticized several US states for reopening their economies despite the rising number of infections.
- Former Director of the US Centers for Disease Control Tom Frieden has advocated an expansion of testing in the United States, warning that the pandemic will be "long and difficult."
- The European Commissioner for Economy, Paolo Gentiloni, has predicted that the European Union will face an economic recession this year with a decline in economic output of more than seven percent.
- Dutch Prime Minister Mark Rutte has announced the easing lockdown restrictions over a period of four months. Rutte also announced that recreational golf and tennis would be allowed from 11 May but organised sports would resume from 1 September.
- French vaccines subsidiary Sanofi Pasteur has announced that it is planning to test an experimental vaccine developing in partnership with the British company GlaxoSmithKline.
- The German Government has announced that Germany's football league Bundesliga will resume matches from 15 May.
- Russian Culture Minister Olga Lyubimova has tested positive for the coronavirus. Russian President Vladimir Putin has

warned against rushing to lift lockdown measures, warning that doing so would undo efforts to combat COVID-19.

- The Slovakian Government has reopened several businesses, including restaurant terraces, hotels, and shops outside of shopping malls. The Government has allowed weddings and religious services to take place in limited numbers.
- Spain's parliament, the Cortes Generales, has extended the country's state of emergency by two weeks.
- Turkish Health Minister Fahrettin Koca has announced plans to reopen the economy, including specifying social distancing and facial mask requirements.
- In the United Kingdom, British epidemiologist Neil Ferguson resigned from the British Government's Scientific Advisory Group for Emergencies (SAGE) after breaching lockdown and social distancing rules by meeting with his married lover.
- UK Prime Minister Boris Johnson has stated that the British Government will announce its plan to ease coronavirus lockdown restrictions from Sunday (9 May).
- World Health Organization Director-General Tedros Adhanom urged countries emerging from lockdown to do it "extremely carefully and in a phased approach."
- In China, authorities in the northeastern border town of Suifenhe announced the loosening of restrictions brought in to combat a surge of cases from neighbouring Russia. 120 schools in Wuhan reopened for nearly 60,000 senior high school students.
- In China, authorities in the northeastern border town of Suifenhe announced the loosening of restrictions brought in to combat a surge of cases from neighbouring Russia. 120

schools in Wuhan reopened for nearly 60,000 senior high school students.

- The Indian Government has embarked on efforts to repatriate 400,000 stranded Indian nationals via chartered flights and Indian Navy ships.
- Indonesian President Joko Widodo expressed a sense of urgency to bring the country's COVID-19 pandemic under control and "break the curve" in May. The Indonesian Government has also postponed the country's local elections until December 2020.
- Iranian Ministry of Health and Medical Education spokesperson Kianoush Jahanpour warned COVID-19 cases were rising over the past three to four days due to changes in people's behaviour. Iran had reported 1,680 new cases, bringing the total number to over 100,000.
- Morocco has purchased more drones from Chinese drone manufacture DJI.
- The Pakistani Government became concerned that repatriated Pakistani migrant workers returning from the United Arab Emirates may be carrying the coronavirus.
- Qatar Airways's CEO Akbar Al Baker has announced that the airline would be cutting jobs as a result of the economic fallout of the COVID-19 pandemic.
- The Director-General of the WHO reported that, since the start of April, an average of 80,000 cases of COVID-19 per day had been reported to the WHO.
- The UN Secretary-General launched a new report showing that the COVID-19 pandemic was intensifying inequalities experienced by the world's one billion people with disabilities, calling for an inclusive recovery and response.

- New analysis by the UN Office on Drugs and Crime suggested that coronavirus containment measures were placing victims of human trafficking at risk of further exploitation, including by organized crime networks.

7 May

- Afghanistan has reported a total of 3,563 cases and 106 deaths. Kabul has reported 925 cases, including 346 medical staff.
- The Africa CDC has reported over 50,000 total cases in Africa, with 8,000 in South Africa.
- Belarus has reported a total of 19,225 cases and at least 112 deaths. The Belarussian government has refused to impose any lockdown restrictions and quarantine measures.
- Brazil has reported 10,503 new confirmed cases and 615 deaths.
- China has reported two new cases, bringing the official tally to 82,885. The official death toll stands at 4,633.
- France has reported 178 new cases, bringing the total to 25,987. 23,208 remain in hospital, with 2,961 in intensive care.
- India has reported 3,561 new cases, bringing the total to 52,952. Indian authorities have reported 1,783 deaths.
- Indonesia has reported 338 new cases, bringing the total to 12,776. 35 have died, bringing the death toll to 930. 96,717 people have been tested, and 2,381 have recovered.
- Italy has reported 274 deaths, bringing the death toll to 29,958. Italy has reported 1,401 new cases, bringing the total to 215,858.
- Latvia has reported a total of 909 cases and 18 deaths.

- Malaysia has reported 39 new cases, bringing the total number to 6,467. 74 patients have been discharged, bringing the total number of recovered to 4,776. 1,584 remain hospitalised, with 19 in intensive care and 18 on ventilator support. The death toll remains at 107.
- Mexico has reported a total of 27,634 cases and 2,704 deaths.
- The Netherlands has reported 455 cases, bringing the total to 41,774. Dutch health authorities have reported 84 new deaths, bringing the death toll to 5,288.
- New Zealand has reported one new case, bringing the total to 1,489 (1,139 confirmed and 350 probable). Health authorities have also reported 16 new recoveries, bringing the total to 1,332. A record 7,323 tests were completed the day before.
- Qatar has reported 918 new cases, bringing the total to 16,592. The death toll remains at 12.
- Russia has reported 11,231 new cases (6,703 in Moscow), bringing the total to 177,160 (92,676 in Moscow). Russia has also reported 88 new deaths, bringing the death toll to 1,625. Mayor of Moscow Sergei Sobyanin has claimed that the number of cases in Moscow is much higher than the official figures.
- Singapore has reported 741 new cases, bringing the total to 20,939.
- Spain has reported 213 deaths, bringing the death toll to 26,070. Spain has reported a total of 221,447 cases.
- Thailand has reported three new cases, bringing the total to 2,992.

- Turkey has reported 57 new deaths, bringing the death toll to 3,641. Turkey has also reported 1,977 new cases, bringing the total to 133,721.
- Ukraine has reported 507 new cases and 13 new deaths, bringing the total numbers to 13,691 and 340, respectively; a total of 2,396 patients have recovered.
- The United Kingdom has reported 539 new deaths, bringing the death toll to 30,615.
- The government confirms that 400,000 gowns ordered from Turkey to protect NHS staff from coronavirus have been impounded after failing to meet the required safety standards.
- The Bank of England warns that the economy is on course to shrink by 14% in 2020 because of the impact of COVID-19, pushing the UK into its deepest recession on record.
- Baroness Dido Harding, chair of NHS Improvement and former CEO of TalkTalk is appointed to lead the government's programme of testing and tracing, supported by John Newton of Public Health England. Testing will be led by Sarah-Jane Marsh, chief executive of Birmingham Women's and Children's Hospitals, and tracing will be led by Tom Riordan, chief executive of Leeds City Council.
- The UK stages another round of applause for NHS staff and key workers, the seventh to be held on consecutive Thursdays at 8 pm.
- The United States has reported its first death in immigration custody. Carlos Ernestor Escobar died from complications related to COVID-19 in a San Diego immigration detention facility.

- Brazilian Health Minister Nelson Teich stated during a media conference that lockdowns were likely necessary. In addition, over 20 Brazilian government officials, including spokesperson Otavio Rego Barros, communications chief Fabio Wajngarten and Secretary of Institutional Security Augusto Heleno, have tested positive for COVID-19.
- Canadian Prime Minister Justin Trudeau has announced that the federal government and ten provinces will be supplementing the pay of essential workers, including those working in rest homes. Trudeau confirmed that the federal government will contribute C$4 billion, which accounted for 75% of the total cost.
- El Salvador suspended public transportation for 15 days.
- The Mexican Government has converted the former presidential residence Los Pinos into a temporary home for health workers battling COVID-19. 58 doctors and workers are staying at the facility, which can house 100 people.
- United States President Donald Trump and Vice President Mike Pence have tested negative for the coronavirus after a US military serviceman who worked in the White House was infected with the coronavirus. Trump mentioned that Russian President Vladimir Putin accepted a shipment of ventilators from the United States.
- United States federal judge Douglas P. Woodlock has overturned Governor of Massachusetts Charlie Baker's order designating gun shops "non-essential businesses," arguing that closing them down for the duration of the coronavirus pandemic violated the Second Amendment. As a result, gunshops in the state are allowed to reopen. New York state authorities have extended a moratorium on evictions for non-

payment of rent by another 60 days until 20 August in order to combat the spread of COVID-19.

- Washington state officials have advised people against holding "COVID-19 parties".
- The Coordinating Body of Indigenous Peoples of the Amazon Basin has launched an Amazon Emergency Fund to raise funds to protect 3 million Amazon rainforest inhabitants from the effects of the coronavirus.
- The International Monetary Fund has approved a total of US$18 billion in aid requests from 50 of its 189 members. IMF spokesperson Gerry Rice also confirmed that the IMF was processing requests for aid from over 50 countries, including South Africa, Sri Lanka, and Zambia.
- United Nations Under-Secretary-General for Humanitarian Affairs and Emergency Relief Coordinator Mark Lowcock has appealed for US$4.7 billion in funding to top up its US$2 billion funds to help developing countries combat COVID-19.
- The United States airliner Frontier Airlines has announced that it will begin testing the temperatures of all crew and passengers from 1 June, barring entry to anyone with a temperature over 100.4 degrees Fahrenheit (38 Celsius).
- Dr. John Nkengasong, the head of the Africa Centres for Disease Control and Prevention (Africa CDC), has rejected assertions by Tanzanian President John Magufuli that his country's COVID-19 tests are unreliable. The tests were supplied by the Africa CDC and the Jack Ma Foundation.
- Indian health authorities have identified a new cluster in the Koyambedu market in Chennai, which has been linked to 500 cases in Tamil Nadu and the adjacent Kerala states. Indian authorities are contacting tracing and quarantining

7,000 people who visited the market. Areas with high numbers of COVID-19 cases include Mumbai, New Delhi, and Ahmedabad.

- Chinese Foreign Ministry spokesperson Hua Chunying reiterated Beijing's support for WHO's efforts to combat the COVID-19 pandemic. She criticised the US and other countries for "politicising" the issue and accused US Secretary of State Mike Pompeo of spreading lies about China.
- Japanese Economy Minister Yasutoshi Nishimura said that restrictions could be lifted in areas where infection rates have declined. That same day, the Japanese Government approved Gilead Sciences' remdesivir as a treatment for COVID-19.
- New Zealand Sport and Recreation Minister Grant Robertson announced that professional sports will resume domestically next week under COVID-19 Alert Level 2 with the necessary public health measures in place.
- Egyptian Prime Minister Mostafa Madbouly has extended the country's nighttime curfew until the end of Ramadan.
- Pakistani President Imran Khan announced that Pakistan will be lifting lockdown restrictions on 9 May , despite rising case numbers due to the adverse economic impact on workers.
- The Danish Government has allowed the entire retail sector, including shopping malls, to reopen from 11 May. Restaurants and cafes will reopen one week later.
- French Prime Minister Edouard Philippe has announced that France will be relaxing COVID-19 lockdown restrictions from 11 May but some restrictions would remain in Paris due to several new cases. French Interior Minister Christophe

Castaner confirmed that the country's borders will remain closed despite the planned lifting of the nationwide lockdown on 11 May.

- German Chancellor Angela Merkel stated during a media interview that the coronavirus pandemic could last for a year. Yesterday, Merkel had announced steps to ease Germany's lockdown while launching an "emergency break mechanism" in the event of a resurgence of the pandemic. The Robert Koch Institute has estimated that the coronavirus' reproduction rate is 0.65, meaning that 100 people who contracted the disease infect on average 65, suggesting that the rate of infection is declining. A senior German health official Lars Schaade also warned that a second COVID-19 wave was possible depending on people's behaviour and compliance with health and social distancing regulations.
- Germany's football league Bundesliga has announced that professional and second division matches will resume on 16 May.
- Georgian Prime Minister Giorgi Gakharia has announced that the Georgian Government will lift the lockdown in Tbilisi and allow shops to reopen on 11 May. The lockdown on Rustavi will be lifted on 14 May. Domestic tourism will be resumed on 15 June while foreign tourists will be allowed into the country from 1 July. The country remains in a state of emergency until 22 May, which includes a night curfew, the closure of non-essential businesses, and a ban on gatherings of more than three people.
- The Icelandic Government has eased coronavirus lockdown restrictions by allowing gatherings of up to 50 people and letting children's activities return to normal.

- Italian Prime Minister Giuseppe Conte and Roman Catholic Church Archbishop Gualtiero Bassetti have signed an agreement to allow Italian Catholics to attend Mass from 18 May, ending a dispute between the two parties. Under lockdown restrictions, the Government had not allowed Masses as part of its ban on public gatherings. Italian priests will determine the number of people allowed into churches, and churches may hold multiple services to comply with social distancing requirements.
- Latvian Prime Minister Krisjanis Karins has announced that Latvia will allow public gatherings of 25 people from 12 May as part of efforts to ease the lockdown.
- In the Netherlands, Health Minister Hugo de Jonge clarified that spectators could not attend sports arenas until a vaccine for the coronavirus had been developed.
- Norwegian Prime Minister Erna Solberg has announced that Norway will be reopening by mid-June, citing the country's success in containing the COVID-19 pandemic.
- The Polish governing coalition has postponed the 2020 Polish presidential election due to the COVID-19 pandemic. Poland's lower legislature, the Sejm, has passed government-sponsored legislation allowing the presidential election to resume by postal vote.
- In Russia, the Mayor of Moscow Sergei Sobyanin has extended the city's lockdown restrictions until 31 May. In the United Kingdom, a study by a team of University College London researchers Dr. Rob Aldridge and Dr. Delan Devakumar published in Wellcome Open Research found that the risk of dying from COVID-19 was 3.24 times higher for Black Africans, 2.41 times higher for British

Bangladeshis, 2.21 times higher for Black Caribbeans and 1.7 times higher for British Indians compared to the general population. Their study drew upon National Health Service data of 16,272 patients who had died from COVID-19 between 1 March and 21 April. The study's findings were endorsed by the British Government's Office for National Statistics.

- A spokesperson for British Prime Minister Boris Johnson announced that the UK Government will announce a limited easing of the country's lockdown restrictions next week. Organisers have postponed the 2020 Notting Hill Carnival due to the COVID-19 pandemic. Foreign Secretary Dominic Raab has opposed easing the country's lockdown, warning that doing so could lead to an increase in infection rates. Similarly, Deputy First Minister of Northern Ireland Michelle O'Neill has announced that Northern Ireland does not intend to lift coronavirus pandemic restrictions.
- Secretary of State for Northern Ireland Brandon Lewis acknowledged that UK health authorities were unable to use 400,000 medical gowns imported from Turkey since they did not meet British standards.
- The United Nations Office on Drugs and Crime issued a statement noting that coronavirus-related restrictions have pushed up the price of illicit drugs.

8 May

- Argentina has reported a total of over 5,611 cases and 293 deaths.
- Australia has reported a total of under 7,000 cases and nearly 100 deaths. 800 people remain in the hospital.

- Brazil has reported 10,222 new cases, bringing the total to 145,328. Brazil has reported 751 deaths, bringing the death toll to 9,897.
- China has reported one new case and 15 new asymptomatic cases. China has officially recorded a total of 82,887 cases, 78,000 recoveries, and 4,633 deaths.
- France has reported 243 deaths, raising the death toll to 26,230. 2,868 remain in intensive care.
- The six members of the Gulf Cooperation Council have reported a total of almost 80,000 cases and 486 deaths.
- Honduras has reported a total of 1,461 cases and 99 deaths.
- Italy has reported 243 deaths, bringing the death toll to 30,201.
- Malaysia has reported 68 new cases, bringing the total number to 6,535. 1,564 remain in hospital, with 17 in intensive care and seven on ventilator support. Malaysian authorities have discharged 88 patients, bringing the number of recovered to 4,864. The death toll remains at 107.
- New Zealand has reported one new confirmed case while a previous probable case was reclassified as confirmed, bringing the total to 1,490 (1,141 confirmed and 349 probable). 15 new recoveries have been reported, bringing the total to 1,347, or 90% of all cases. A record 7,812 tests were completed the previous day.
- Qatar has reported 1,311 new cases, bringing the total to over 20,000. Most of these cases have occurred among foreign migrant workers. The country has reported 12 deaths.

- Russia has reported 10,699 new cases, bringing the total to 187,859. Russia has reported 98 deaths, bringing the death toll to 1,723.
- Singapore has reported 768 new cases, bringing the total to 21,707.
- Spain has reported 229 new deaths, bringing the death toll to 26,229. The country also reported a total of 222,857 cases.
- Thailand has reported eight new cases, bringing the total to 3,000. The death toll remains at 55.
- In the UK, the death of a six-week-old baby is reported.
- With the UK beginning another Bank Holiday weekend, Environment Secretary George Eustice urges the public to abide by the rules of the lockdown restrictions and warns people to have to be "realistic" about the loosening of the measures.
- Ukraine has reported 504 new cases and 21 new deaths, bringing the total numbers to 14,195 and 361 respectively; a total of 2,706 patients have recovered.
- In the United States, New York has reported that 73 children have been infected with a new inflammatory syndrome believed to be linked to COVID-19. One five-year-old boy has reportedly died.
- Yemen has reported nine new cases, bringing the total to 34. Yemen has reported two deaths, bringing the death toll to seven.
- In Mexico, some local authorities have ordered the closing of markets, pasty, and flower shops for the duration of Mother's Day.

- The White House confirmed that a member of Vice-President Mike Pence's staff has tested positive for the coronavirus. Pence also called for a resumption of religious services while speaking at a Presbyterian Church in Des Moines, Iowa. In addition, the White House spokesperson Kayleigh McEnany announced that White House Coronavirus Task Force coordinator Dr. Deborah Birx would be advising the US Government on the distribution of Gilead Sciences' new remdesivir drug.
- The United States Department of Labor has reported that the unemployment rate reached 14.7% in April, with an estimated 20.5 million jobs lost as a result of the COVID-19 pandemic. This figure exceeds the unemployment rate caused by the late 2000s Great Recession.
- The United States Government has blocked a vote at the United Nations Security Council on a resolution relating to the COVID-19 pandemic due to its reference to the World Health Organization.
- The US Food and Drug Administration has revoked US authorization for face masks produced by more than 60 manufacturers on the grounds that they failed to meet health and safety standards for health workers.
- The Associated Press has reported that several US state governors have been "disregarding or creatively interpreting" White House safety guidelines for businesses.
- Many of Facebook's employees will be allowed to work remotely until the end of 2020. Most of Facebook's offices are closed until 6 July.

- Global tech giant Apple Inc. has announced that it will be reopening its retail stores in the United States from next week.
- The United Food and Commercial Workers International Union (UFCW) has announced its opposition to reopening US meatpacking plants, citing concerns for worker safety.
- Also, in the United States, the annual Miss America pageant commemorating its centennial anniversary was originally scheduled for December. It was canceled and included associated state pageants due to be held in the upcoming summer, marking the first time since 1934 to cancel the pageant.
- President of South Africa Cyril Ramaphosa has announced that parole will be granted to 19,000 low-risk prisoners in response to a United Nations call for governments to reduce prison populations in order to allow social distancing and self-isolation.
- Tanzania has received its first shipment of the untested "COVID-Organics" herbal remedy from Madagascar. The World Health Organization has cautioned against using the untested remedy.
- The updated UN Global Humanitarian Response Plan, backed by the WFP and other agencies, sought nearly $7 billion to protect the lives of millions of people and halt the transmission of COVID-19 in over 60 of the world's most fragile countries.
- A new UN Office of Drugs and Crime report on drug market trends during the coronavirus crisis suggested that countries' coronavirus prevention measures had led to the widespread

disruption of trafficking routes for illegal drugs, increasing some prices.

- Dr. John Nkengasong, the head of the Africa Centres for Disease Control and Prevention (Africa CDC), has rejected assertions by Tanzanian President John Magufuli that his country's COVID-19 tests are not reliable. The tests were supplied by the Africa CDC and the Jack Ma Foundation.
- Tanzania has received its first shipment of the untested "COVID-Organics" herbal remedy from Madagascar. The World Health Organization has cautioned against using the untested remedy.
- Argentina has reported a total of over 5,611 cases and 293 deaths.
- Australia has reported a total of under 7,000 cases and nearly 100 deaths. 800 people remain in the hospital.
- Brazil has reported 10,222 new cases, bringing the total to 145,328. Brazil has reported 751 deaths, bringing the death toll to 9,897.
- China has reported one new case and 15 new asymptomatic cases. China has officially recorded a total of 82,887 cases, 78,000 recoveries, and 4,633 deaths.
- The Canadian Province Of Ontario is reporting 477 new cases.
- France has reported 243 deaths, raising the death toll to 26,230. 2,868 remain in intensive care.
- The six members of the Gulf Cooperation Council have reported a total of almost 80,000 cases and 486 deaths.
- Honduras has reported a total of 1,461 cases and 99 deaths.
- Italy has reported 243 deaths, bringing the death toll to 30,201.

- Malaysia has reported 68 new cases, bringing the total number to 6,535. 1,564 remain in hospital, with 17 in intensive care and seven on ventilator support. Malaysian authorities have discharged 88 patients, bringing the number of recovered to 4,864. The death toll remains at 107.
- New Zealand has reported one new confirmed case while a previous probable case was reclassified as confirmed, bringing the total to 1,490 (1,141 confirmed and 349 probable). 15 new recoveries have been reported, bringing the total to 1,347, or 90% of all cases. A record 7,812 tests were completed the previous day.
- Qatar has reported 1,311 new cases, bringing the total to over 20,000. Most of these cases have occurred among foreign migrant workers. The country has reported 12 deaths.
- Russia has reported 10,699 new cases, bringing the total to 187,859. Russia has reported 98 deaths, bringing the death toll to 1,723.
- Singapore has reported 768 new cases, bringing the total to 21,707.
- Spain has reported 229 new deaths, bringing the death toll to 26,229. The country also reported a total of 222,857 cases.
- Thailand has reported eight new cases, bringing the total to 3,000. The death toll remains at 55.
- Ukraine has reported 504 new cases and 21 new deaths, bringing the total numbers to 14,195 and 361 respectively; a total of 2,706 patients have recovered.
- In the United States, New York has reported that 73 children have been infected with a new inflammatory syndrome

believed to be linked to COVID-19. One five-year-old boy has reportedly died.

- Yemen has reported nine new cases, bringing the total to 34. Yemen has reported two deaths, bringing the death toll to seven.
- The European Commission has announced that it will distribute 10 million masks to health workers across the European Union and the United Kingdom. The commission announced that 1.5 million masks will be sent to 17 member states and the UK. The rest will be delivered in weekly installments over the next few weeks. That same day, the European Commission also supported maintaining travel restrictions for another 30 days in order to limit the spread of COVID-19. In addition, the European Commission allowed European governments to assist companies hit by the economic fallout of the coronavirus pandemic by acquiring stakes in the firms, which will be subject to a ban on dividends, share buybacks, bonuses, and acquisitions.
- World War Two commemoration services and parades throughout Europe have been scaled down due to social distancing restrictions and limitations on mass gatherings. German Chancellor Angela Merkel and German President Frank-Walter Steinmeier have laid wreaths at a service in Berlin marking the 75th anniversary of the end of World War Two. French President Emmanuel Macron attended an event at Champs-Elysees. In the United Kingdom, street parades by veterans were cancelled.
- Scientists based at the Vlaams Instituut Voor Biotechnologie in Ghent, Belgium, and the University of Texas, Austin are working to develop an anti-viral treatment based on llama antibodies.

- Germany's Federal Intelligence Service has disputed allegations by US Vice President Mike Pence that the coronavirus originated in a Chinese laboratory, adding that the accusations are an attempt to divert attention away from US efforts to contain the virus.
- The Germany chapter of the Fridays for Future staged a protest outside the Hamburg City Hall while observing strict social distancing measures.
- Ireland's Central Statistics Office has recorded that the country's unemployment rate rose to 28.2% in late April. This figure includes those receiving the emergency coronavirus jobless benefit, which accounts for 5.4%.
- The Malaysian Department of Statistics has released findings showing that 42.5% of companies will need at least six months to recover from the lockdown restrictions, which were lifted on 4 May. The Statistics Department also reported the country's retail sales fell 5.7% to a seven-year low in March 2020.
- The UN High Commissioner for Human Rights Michelle Bachelet warned that some parties to the conflict in Syria, including ISIL terrorist fighters, maybe using the COVID-19 pandemic as "an opportunity to regroup and inflict violence on the population."
- The UN Secretary-General made a global appeal calling for concerted global action to quash the "tsunami" of hate speech accompanying the COVID-19 pandemic.
- UN ECOSOC warned that the COVID-19 outbreak could trigger a humanitarian catastrophe in Haiti.

- The Director-General of the WHO stated that the lessons learned from the eradication of smallpox four decades previously could be applied to the coronavirus pandemic.
- Dr. Peter Embarek, Food Safety and Zoonosis Expert at WHO confirmed that a now-closed Wuhan city wholesale market "played a role" in the outbreak, though it was unclear if it was the original source.
- Australian Prime Minister Scott Morrison announced the easing of social distancing measures as part of a three-stage process to eliminate most restrictions by July 2020 and to get 1 million people back to work. Morrison also clarified that Australian states and territories would decide when to implement each stage, which will be separated by a four-week transition. Treasurer Josh Frydenberg estimated that the lockdown was costing the Australian economy A$4 billion (US$2.6 billion) a week. At the same time, the Reserve Bank of Australia warned that the Australian economy could contract by 10% as a result of the COVID-19 pandemic.
- Chinese Foreign Ministry spokesperson Hua Chunying announced that the Chinese Government supports a review of WHO's response to the COVID-19 pandemic at an "appropriate time" after the pandemic is over.
- Hong Kong allowed gyms, bars, beauty parlours, and cinemas to reopen as part of a relaxation of social distancing measures. A team of Hong Kong researchers led by Dr. Michael Chan Chi-Wai have identified the eyes as an important route for the SARS-CoV-2 virus to enter the human body. The study, published in The Lancet Respiratory Medicine, also found that the coronavirus was more infectious than SARS and the bird flu.

- The Korea Centers for Disease Control and Prevention (Korea CDC) Director Jeong Eun-kyeong announced it was investigating a cluster of outbreaks linked to nightclubs in the capital Seoul's Itaewon neighbourhood.
- Japanese Prime Minister Shinzo Abe and US President Donald Trump agreed to cooperate to develop COVID-19 vaccines and drugs and rejuvenate their economies. The Japanese Ministry of Health, Labour, and Welfare lowered the temperature-related criteria for COVID-19 testing, allowing a wider range of people to check whether they are infected with COVID-19. Previously, only those who had a fever of 37.5 Celsius (99.5 Fahrenheit) or more for four consecutive days could access testing.
- WHO food safety and animal diseases expert Peter Ben Embarek called for more research into Wuhan's Huanan Seafood Wholesale Market's role as an "amplifying setting" in the COVID-19 pandemic.
- Afghan Health Minister Ferozuddin Feroz tests positive for the coronavirus.
- Kuwait has imposed a 20–day total curfew between 4 pm local time on 10 May and 30 May in order to combat the spread of COVID-19.
- The Lebanese Government has eased lockdown restrictions imposed in March, allowing mosques to reopen. However, mosques will have to adhere to social distancing rules.
- UNRWA has launched an emergency appeal to raise US$93.4 million to provide food and cash for vulnerable Palestinians over the next three months.
- President of South Africa Cyril Ramaphosa has announced that parole will be granted to 19,000 low-risk prisoners in

response to a United Nations call for governments to reduce prison populations in order to allow social distancing and self-isolation.

9 May

- Australia reported a total of 6,927 cases and 97 deaths.
- Belarus has recorded a total of 21,101 cases and 26 deaths.
- Canada has reported 157 new deaths, bringing the death toll to 4,628. Canada has reported 1,381 cases, bringing the total to 66,780.
- France has reported 80 deaths, bringing the death toll to 26,310. 22,614 remain in hospital, with 2,812 in intensive care.
- Germany has reported 1,251 cases, bringing the total to 168,551. Germany has reported 147 deaths, bringing the death toll to 7,369.
- Indonesia has reported 533 new cases, bringing the total to 13,645. Indonesia has reported 16 deaths, bringing the total to 959.
- Iran has reported 1,529 new cases, bringing the total to 106,220. Iran has reported 48 deaths, bringing the death toll to 6,589. While most provinces have seen a drop in cases, cases have continued to rise in Khuzestan.
- Italy has reported 194 deaths, bringing the death toll to 30,395. Italy has reported 1,083 new cases, bringing the total to 218,268. 1,034 remain in intensive care.
- Malaysia has reported 54 new cases, bringing the total to 6,589. Malaysia has reported 1 death, bringing the total to 108.

- New Zealand has reported two new cases (one confirmed and the other probable), bringing the total to 1,492 (1,142 confirmed and 350 probable). 21 new recoveries have been reported, bringing the total to 1,368.
- The Philippines has reported 147 cases, bringing the total to 10,610. The Philippines has reported 8 deaths, bringing the total to 704.
- Qatar has reported 1,130 cases, bringing the total to 21,331. Qatar has reported 1 death, bringing the death toll to 13.
- Russia has reported 10,817 cases, bringing the total to 198,676. Russia has reported 104 deaths, bringing the death toll to 1,827.
- Singapore has reported 753 new cases, bringing the total to 22,460.
- South Korea has reported 18 new cases, bringing the total to 10,840. The country has reported 256 deaths.
- Spain has reported 721 new cases, bringing the total to 223,578. Spain has also reported 179 deaths, bringing the total to 26,478.
- Thailand has reported four new cases, bringing the total to 3,004. Thailand has also reported 1 death, bringing the death toll to 56.
- Ukraine has reported 515 new cases and 15 new deaths, bringing the total numbers to 14,710 and 376, respectively; a total of 2,909 patients have recovered.
- The United Kingdom has reported 346 deaths, bringing the death toll to 31,587.
- Transport Secretary Grant Shapps announces £2bn of investment to improve walking and cycling, describing it as a

chance for a "once in a generation change" to the way the public travels.

- The United Kingdom Government has informed airlines that it plans to introduce a 14-day quarantine period for people entering the country. Airliners have raised concerns that it would have damaging repercussions on the aviation industry and economy and have called for a "credible exit plan" and weekly review.
- Belarus has held a military parade to commemorate the 75th anniversary of the end of World War II in Europe, drawing large crowds. By contrast, Russian authorities have cancelled the Victory Day celebrations to contain the coronavirus's spread.
- German Chancellor Angela Merkel and Pope Francis agreed on the need to help poor countries during a telephone conversation on the humanitarian and political situation relating to the coronavirus pandemic. Dresden's soccer team, the Dynamo Dresden, have been placed into quarantine after two members tested positive for COVID-19.
- Spanish Prime Minister Pedro Sánchez has called on people to obey social distancing rules as the country prepares to ease lockdown measures on 11 May, warning that "the virus has not disappeared."
- The United States has reported a total of 1,342,329 cases, 79,906 deaths, and 232,821 recoveries. In New York, Governor Andrew Cuomo has announced that three more children have died of an infectious disease linked to COVID-19.
- President of Argentina Alberto Fernandez has extended the capital Buenos Aires' quarantine until 24 May but has

relaxed quarantine restrictions in other parts of the country. Buenos Aires has been under quarantine since 20 March.

- Brazilian Minister of the Economy Paulo Guedes has called on the Supreme Federal Court to reverse state quarantine measures in order to prevent a shortage of basic commodities.
- US President Donald Trump has announced that the US federal government will buy US$3 billion worth of agricultural goods from the agricultural sector, including dairy, meat, and horticulture producers, in order to combat unemployment and a drop in revenue caused by the COVID-19 pandemic.
- Congressmen Eliot Engel, the Democratic chairman of the United States House Committee on Foreign Affairs, Michael McCaul, the House Committee's ranking Republican member, Senator Jim Risch, the Republican chairman of the United States Senate Committee on Foreign Relations, and Senator Bob Menendez, the Senate Committee's ranking Democratic member, have sent a joint letter to nearly 60 "like-minded" countries asking them to support Taiwan's participation in the World Health Organization. These countries have included Canada, Thailand, Japan, Germany, the United Kingdom, Saudi Arabia and Australia.
- White House Deputy Press Secretary Hogan Gidley confirmed that a military official who worked in close proximity to President Donald Trump had tested positive for the coronavirus on Wednesday. He also confirmed that Trump and Vice President Mike Pence have tested negative for the coronavirus.
- Former US President Barack Obama has criticized President Trump's handling of the COVID-19 pandemic in the United States and urged former Obama Administration staff

members to support Democratic presidential nominee Joe Biden.

- President of Sierra Leone Julius Maada Bio has accused the opposition All People's Congress of inciting "terrorist violence" following a surge of violence linked to the country's coronavirus outbreak.
- The Australian states of Victoria and New South Wales indicated the lessening of business restrictions from next week. Queensland announced that it will ease travel and movement restrictions in a three-stage process, commencing 15 May. South Australia announced that it will ease all movement restrictions by 11 May, while Tasmania will allow people to visit national parks and reserves within 30 km of their homes from 11 May. The Australian Capital Territory allowed people to visit each other and public gatherings of ten people. The Northern Territory allowed people to visit parks and reserves from 1 June with plans to reopen all businesses, facilities, and services by 5 June.
- Chinese Communist Party general secretary Xi Jinping sent a letter to Korean Workers' Party chairman Kim Jong-Un, affirming Beijing's support for Pyongyang in combating the COVID-19 pandemic.
- Hong Kong researchers have tested a three-drug cocktail of lopinavir/ritonavir, ribavirin and interferon-beta on 127 patients with mild symptoms associated with COVID-19. The trial found that patients treated with this cocktail recovered faster than patients given just lopinavir-ritonavir.
- South Korean Vice Health Minister Kim Gang lip announced that health authorities are developing plans to share hospital capacities between the capital Seoul and nearby towns to ensure swift transport of patients and that a spike of

infections in one cluster doesn't overwhelm the country's healthcare system. In addition, Seoul authorities have closed 21,000 nightclubs, hostess bars, and discos after 17 cases were linked to a 29-year old clubgoer in the Itaewon neighbourhood.

- In Afghanistan's Ghor Province, six people have been killed clashes during a protest against the alleged mismanagement of aid to alleviate the social and economic effects of the COVID-19 pandemic.
- The Emir of Kuwait Sabah Al-Ahmad Al-Jaber Al-Sabah has warned that the decline in oil prices and the value of investment assets will threaten the country's financial solvency.
- The Sudanese state of Khartoum has extended a curfew for ten more days due to a high number of cases. Authorities have also banned travel between the capital Khartoum and other states.
- President of Sierra Leone Julius Maada Bio has accused the opposition All People's Congress of inciting "terrorist violence" following a surge of violence linked to the country's coronavirus outbreak.

10 May

- Brazil has reported a total of 10,627 deaths and 155,939 cases. However, scientists believe that the real figures are higher due to a lack of widespread testing.
- Canada has reported 100 new deaths, bringing the death toll to 4,728. Canada has reported 1,216 new cases, bringing the total to 66,796.

- China has reported 14 new cases (12 community transmissions and 2 imported); 11 of these cases occurred in Jilin province and one in Hubei.
- France has reported 70 new deaths, bringing the death toll to 26,380. 36 people have been discharged from intensive care, bringing the total number in intensive care down to 2,776.
- Germany has reported 667 new cases, bringing the total to 169,218. Germany has also reported 26 deaths, bringing the death toll to 7,395.
- Iran has reported 51 new deaths.
- Lebanon has reported 36 new cases, bringing the total to 845. Lebanon's death toll remains at 26.
- Malaysia has reported 67 new cases (49 of them foreigners), bringing the total to 6,656. 1,525 remain in hospital; 18 in intensive care and 6 on ventilators. 96 have been discharged, bringing the total number of recoveries to 5,025. The death toll remains at 108.
- New Zealand has reported two new cases (both confirmed), bringing the total to 1,494 (1,144 confirmed and 350 probable). Two people remain in the hospital. Three people have recovered, bringing the total to 1,371.
- The Philippines has reported 184 new cases, bringing the total to 10,794. 15 deaths have been recorded, bringing the death toll to 719. 82 have recovered, bringing the total number of recovered to 1,924.
- Russia has reported 11,012 new cases, bringing the total to 209,668. Russia has reported 88 deaths, bringing the death toll to 1,195.

- Singapore has reported 876 new cases, bringing the total to 23,336. In addition, 33 false-positive tests were recorded due to calibration issues in one of the test kits.
- South Korea has reported 34 new cases (26 community transmissions and eight imported). Most of these cases have been linked to nightclubs in Seoul's Itaewon district.
- Spain has reported 143 deaths, bringing the death toll to 26,621. Spain has reported 224,390 casualties.
- Thailand has reported five new cases, bringing the total to 3,009. The death toll remains at 59.
- Turkey has reported a total of 137,115 cases and 3,739 deaths.
- Ukraine has reported 522 new cases and 15 new deaths, bringing the total numbers to 15,232 and 391, respectively; a total of 2,909 patients have recovered.
- The United Kingdom has reported 269 deaths, bringing the national death toll to 31,855.
- The UK government updates its coronavirus message from "stay at home, protect the NHS, save lives" to "stay alert, control the virus, save lives". The Opposition Labour Party expresses concern the slogan could be confusing, and leaders of the devolved governments in Scotland, Wales and Northern Ireland say they will keep the original slogan.
- A new alert scale system is announced, ranging from green (level one) to red (level five), similar to the UK's Terror Threat Levels.
- A recorded address by Boris Johnson is broadcast at 7pm in which he outlines a "conditional plan" to reopen society, but says it is "not the time simply to end the lockdown this week", and describes the plans as "the first careful steps to

modify our measures". Those who cannot work from home, such as construction workers and manufacturing workers, are encouraged to return to work from the following day but avoid public transport if possible. The guidance on the number of outdoor exercise periods will be lifted from Wednesday 13 May.

- Outlining future easing of restrictions, Johnson says "step two" – no sooner than 1 June – would include reopening some shops and the return of primary school pupils, beginning with reception, Year 1 and Year 6; and that secondary pupils facing exams next year would get some time in school before the summer holiday. "Step three" – at the earliest by July – would begin reopening the hospitality industry and other public places.
- Johnson also says that passengers arriving into the UK on international flights (apart from those from the Republic of Ireland) will soon be asked to go into quarantine for fourteen days.
- In the United States, at least 25,600 residents and workers have died at nursing homes and other long-term care facilities for the elderly. The coronavirus has affected 143,000 people at about 7,500 facilities.
- About 4 million cases, almost 1.4 million recoveries, and over 279,000 deaths have been reported globally.
- The Brazilian National Congress has decreed three days of mourning to mark the 10,000 Brazilians who have died and called on Brazilians to follow health authorities' recommendations in order to reduce infection rates.
- In the United States, several US officials, including Robert Redfield, the Director of the Centers for Disease Control and

Prevention (CDC), Stephen Hahn, the Director of the Food and Drug Administration, and Dr Anthony Fauci, the leader of the White House Coronavirus Task Force, have entered into self-isolation after coming in contact with an individual who tested positive for the coronavirus.

- Governor of New York Andrew Cuomo has required nursing homes in New York to test staff twice a week for COVID-19.
- Tesla CEO and tech entrepreneur Elon Musk has threatened to pull the company's electrical vehicle factory and headquarters out of California and sued Alameda County's health department after health authorities stopped the factory from reopening. Musk has accused Alameda health authorities of overstepping both state and federal regulations.
- The US airline trade group Airlines for America has endorsed allowing the Transportation Security Administration to conduct temperature checks on passengers for the duration of the coronavirus pandemic.
- In Australia, New South Wales Premier Gladys Berejiklian allowed restaurants, playgrounds and outdoor pools to reopen after extensive testing showed that the spread of COVID-19 had slowed sharply. Australian Chief Medical Officer Brendan Murphy dismissed conspiracy theories that COVID-19 is linked to 5G cellular phone technology following an anti-lockdown protest in Melbourne. Protesters had claimed that the COVID-19 pandemic was a government conspiracy to control the global population.
- Djibouti's Foreign Minister Mahamoud Ali Youssouf has announced that the country will be lifting lockdown measures despite the high number of cases in order to allow people to make a living and go to work.

- Iranian authorities reimposed restrictions on Khuzestan province.
- Lebanese Interior Minister Mohammad Fahmi has extended the country's nighttime curfew from 7 pm to 5 am local in response to a surge in cases.
- Montenegrin Prime Minister Dusko Markovic has promoted his country as a "CoronaFree" holiday destination, with the holiday season due to begin on 1 July.
- In Russia, Mayor of Moscow Sergei Sobyanin confirmed that a fire at a Moscow hospital treating patients of the coronavirus had been killed. 200 patients were also evacuated from the hospital.
- The Turkish government has relaxed restrictions on elderly people over the age of 65, allowing them to leave their homes for four hours a day. The government also announced plans to allow young people under the age of 20 to leave their homes later in the week.
- United Kingdom Secretary of State for Transport Grant Shapps has announced that the British Government's coronavirus test and tracing app trial is going well on the Isle of Wight. That same day, British Prime Minister Boris Johnson announced that country's lockdown will remain in place until 1 June while lifting some lockdown restrictions. From 11 May, people will be encouraged to return to work. From 13 May, people will be allowed to exercise for an unlimited time while adhering to social distancing measures.
- Malaysian Prime Minister Muhyiddin Yassin has extended the country's movement control order (MCO) until 9 June, the fourth extension since 18 March. Earlier, the Malaysian government had downgraded lockdown restrictions on 4 May

under a "condition MCO," which allowed certain businesses to resume operations.

11 May

- The UK government publishes a 50-page document setting out further details of the phases for lifting the lockdown restrictions. Boris Johnson gives further details as he makes his first statement on the virus to Parliament.
- Amid concerns about the safety of people returning to work, Johnson tells the Downing Street daily briefing he is not expecting a "sudden big flood" of people returning to work and that companies will have to prove they have introduced safety measures before they can reopen.
- The UK government advises people in England to wear face coverings in enclosed spaces where social distancing is impossible, such as on public transport and in shops.
- Air passengers arriving on flights from France will also be exempt from new quarantine rules.
- Sir David Norgrove, chair of the UK Statistics Authority, writes to Matt Hancock seeking clarity on the targets for the number of tests and the reporting of the number carried out each day.
- Teaching unions express their concern at government plans to reopen schools on 1 June, describing them as "reckless" and unsafe.
- Fertility clinics can apply to the Human Fertilisation and Embryology Authority to reopen.
- Malaysia has reported 70 new cases, bringing the total to 6,726. There are 1,504 active cases, with 20 cases in intensive care. 88 have been discharged, bringing the total

number of recovered to 5,113. Malaysia has reported 1 new death, bringing the death toll to 109.

- New Zealand has reported three new cases (all confirmed), bringing the total to 1,497 (1,147 confirmed and 350 probable). 15 new recoveries have been reported, bringing the total to 1,386. The number of active cases has dropped below 90.
- Singapore has reported 486 new cases, bringing the total to 23,822. Subsequently, 35 false-positive results were subtracted from the tally, bringing the total to 23,787. Another death was later confirmed, bringing the death toll to 21, with another who died from a heart attack and subsequently tested positive.
- Ukraine has reported 416 new cases and 17 new deaths, bringing the total numbers to 15,648 and 408, respectively; a total of 3,288 patients have recovered.
- New Zealand Prime Minister Jacinda Ardern announced that the country will downgrade its lockdown to alert level 2 from 14 May, lifting lockdown restrictions while maintaining physical distancing in public and private gatherings with more than ten people. Schools could reopen on 18 May, while bars (defined as on-licence premises which primarily serve beverages) could reopen on 21 May. A decision will be made on 25 May on whether to raise the ten–people limit on private gatherings.
- South Korean President Moon Jae-in urged citizens not to lower their guard but has urged calm amid an infection cluster around Seoul's Itaewon's neighbourhood.
- WHO Director-General Tedros Adhanom Ghebreyesus warned the resurgence of COVID-19 cases in South Korea,

China, and Germany following stay-at-home restrictions, indicating their complexity.

- UN ECOSOC held a wide-ranging policy discussion, "Joining Forces: Effective Policy Solutions for Covid-19 Response", stressing a range of multilateral solutions while also committing to getting back on track for the Sustainable Development Goals.
- Three senior UN officials in the Middle East, including UNICEF and the UN Human Rights Office, jointly called for the release of Palestinian children from Israeli-run prisons and detentions centres due to the risk of COVID-19 infection.
- The head of UNAIDS warned that two decades of treatment gains were under threat due to the pandemic.

12 May

- The Canadian province of Ontario has reported 361 new cases.
- In the United Kingdom, figures released by the Office for National Statistics and the devolved administrations indicate the death toll from COVID-19 exceeds 40,000 – including almost 11,000 care home residents – although week-by-week numbers continue to fall. In care homes in England and Wales, the year-to-date COVID-19 total reaches 8,312, but the weekly number (to 1 May) shows a decrease for the first time since the start of the pandemic.
- Chancellor Rishi Sunak extends the UK's furlough scheme until October, with employees receiving 80% of their monthly wages up to £2,500. A quarter of the workforce, some 7.5 million people, are now covered by the scheme, costing £14bn a month.

- India has reported 87 deaths and 3,604 new cases, bringing the total number of cases to 70,756.
- Malaysia has reported 16 more cases, bringing the total number to 6,742. 110 patients have recovered, bringing the total number to 5,223. The death toll remains at 109.
- New Zealand has reported no new cases, with the total remaining at 1,497 (1,147 confirmed and 350 probable). 12 new recoveries have been reported, bringing the total number of recoveries to 1,398.
- Singapore has reported 884 new cases, bringing the total to 24,671. Two more deaths from other causes were recorded, subsequently tested positive.
- Ukraine has reported 375 new cases and 17 new deaths, bringing the total numbers to 16,023 and 425, respectively; a total of 3,373 patients have recovered.
- Despite Brazil recording its highest daily death toll with 881 fatalities so far, President Jair Bolsonaro stated his intent to push for the reopening of non-essential businesses such as gyms and hair salons amidst strong resistance from state governors. Brazil has recorded over 12,400 coronavirus deaths, the sixth-highest total in the world.
- In the United States, House Speaker Nancy Pelosi unveiled the Democrat Party's $3 trillion pandemic relief proposal, with aid for struggling states and another round of $1,200 direct payments to American families, as well as a $25 billion bailout to the Postal Service, and $3.6 billion to ensure election security. Republican Senators immediately rejected the proposal, determining it to be 'too large and far-reaching'.

- US Republican Senators have proposed legislation enabling Donald Trump to apply sanctions to China if the country does not provide a 'full accounting' for the origins of the coronavirus. Senator Jim Inhofe stated that "The Chinese Communist Party must be held accountable for the detrimental role in this pandemic. Their outright deception of the origin and spread of the virus cost the world valuable time and lives as it began to spread".
- The British Transport Police have launched an investigation into the death of London railway ticket office worker Belly Mujinga, who became ill after being spat upon by a man who claimed that he had COVID-19 on 22 March 2020. The Transport Salaried Staffs Association had highlighted Mujinga's death to draw attention to transport staff's dangerous working conditions and lack of personal protective equipment.
- UNICEF warned that as the coronavirus outbreak entered its fifth month, the health crisis was "quickly becoming a child rights crisis", requesting $1.6 billion to support its humanitarian response for children affected by the pandemic, as without it, an additional 6,000 under-fives could die daily.
- In an online meeting with religious leaders via the UN Alliance of Civilizations, the UN Secretary-General noted the coronavirus pandemic revealed "our common humanity", stressing the important role that religious leaders could play in limiting the damage caused by COVID-19.
- Indian Prime Minister Narendra Modi has announced an economic stimulus package worth $266 billion, equivalent to 10% of India's GDP, to support the economy during the

coronavirus pandemic, largely praised by investors and economists around the world.

13 May

- The Canadian province of Ontario has reported 329 new cases.
- Indonesia has reported 689 new cases, bringing the cases to 15,438. 21 have died, bringing the death toll to 1,028. 3,287 have recovered.
- Lesotho has reported its first case.
- The Health Protection (Coronavirus, Restrictions) (England) (Amendment No. 2) Regulations 2020 (SI 500) come into effect, allowing the reopening of garden centres, sports courts and recycling centres. In addition to outdoor exercise, open-air recreation is also permitted with no more than one member of another household. Government announcements gloss these with the (non-enforceable) requirement that social distancing must be practised. House moves and viewings are also permitted.
- After figures indicate the UK economy shrank by 2% in the first three months of 2020 and is shrinking at the fastest rate since the late 2000s global recession, Chancellor Rishi Sunak says it is "very likely" the country is in a "significant recession".
- Creamfields, scheduled for 27–30 August, announces the cancellation of the 2020 edition due to the pandemic.
- Malaysia has reported 37 new cases (four imported and 33 local transmissions), bringing the total to 6,779. 58 have recovered, bringing the total number of recoveries to 5,281.

Malaysia has reported 2 deaths, bringing the death toll to 111.

- New Zealand has reported no new cases, with the total number of cases remaining at 1,497. NZ authorities have also reported four recoveries, bringing the total to 1,402.
- Singapore has reported 675 new cases, bringing the total to 25,346.
- Ukraine has reported 402 new cases and 14 new deaths, bringing the total numbers to 16,425 and 439, respectively; a total of 3,716 patients have recovered.
- In Peru, President Martin Vizcarra stated that the coronavirus had 'peaked' in the country, whilst also confirming that Peru would move into the final stage of lockdown, two months after the first confirmed case in the country. Although the lockdown is due to end on 24 May, social distancing will still be enforced in public spaces.
- In the United States, cab companies Uber and Lyft now require passengers to wear masks.
- The American Federal Reserve Chair Jerome Powell warned of a recession resulting from the coronavirus pandemic and urged the White House and Congress to take preventative measures. Powell cautioned that business bankruptcies and unemployment for millions of Americans will remain a serious economic risk.
- President of South Africa Cyril Ramaphosa has said that his government will begin talks on moving most of the country from "alert level 4" to "alert level 3" by the end of May, although areas with the highest rates of infection would remain at "alert level 4".

- Chinese authorities in Wuhan announce preparations for testing all 11 million residents after six new cases were confirmed at the weekend.
- The New Zealand Government passed the COVID-19 Public Health Response Bill, which allows police to enter homes without a warrant to enforce lockdown restrictions despite opposition from the National and ACT parties and the Human Rights Commission. The government also lifted the country's state of emergency, revised level 2 restrictions to allow people to attend funerals and tangihanga, and shifted NCEA high school exams from 6 November to 16 November.
- The German Interior Minister Horst Seehofer announces the country's plans for free travel in Europe by 15 June. Restrictions on the Austrian border will be eased on 15 May to allow business trips and family visits. The Austrian government also announced that there are plans in place to reopen the Austrian-German border in mid-June.
- The Irish Taoiseach Leo Varadkar has said that Ireland may introduce a mandatory quarantine for arriving international travellers, rather than the current system whereby the quarantine is only advised. This comes days after the British government announced plans for a similar measure.
- Polish Prime Minister Mateusz Morawiecki has announced that Poland will reopen hairdressers and restaurants from 18 May and return students in the first three years of school.
- Professor Albert Rizvanov, director of the Clinical Research Centre for Precision and Regenerative Medicine at Russia's Kazan Federal University, claimed that hot weather does not kill COVID-19, despite earlier claims that the virus could not

survive temperatures above 36 °C. This comes as Russia confirmed more than 10,000 new cases in a day. Russia suspended the use of a certain brand of Russian-manufactured ventilators that have caused two fires.

- The Turkish government's economic stimulus to support businesses during the pandemic has reached $34 billion, equivalent to 5% of the Turkish GDP, Finance Minister Berat Albayrak has said.
- In England, the first easing of lockdown restrictions occurred, with people being allowed outside for unlimited exercise and essential businesses being encouraged to reopen. These restrictions only applied to England, with the other parts of the UK remaining under a tighter lockdown. Public Health England approved a coronavirus antibody test kit manufactured by Swiss company Roche Holdings AG after it was found to be close to 100% accurate.
- Lebanon is examining the possibility of obtaining financial aid via the International Monetary Fund to protect the country's struggling economy, significantly worsened by coronavirus restrictions. The country first asked the IMF for assistance on 1 May.
- Emirates, the national airline of the United Arab Emirates, has announced plans to resume some scheduled flight operations from 21 May. In Dubai, public parks and private beaches are permitted to reopen.
- President of South Africa Cyril Ramaphosa has said that his government will begin talks on moving most of the country from "alert level 4" to "alert level 3" by the end of May, although areas with the highest rates of infection would remain at "alert level 4".

- In its World Economic Situation and Prospect report update, the UN Department of Economic and Social Affairs (DESA) reported that as of mid-2020, the gross domestic product (GDP) in developed countries would plunge to -5.0 per cent. In comparison, the output of developing countries would shrink by 0.7 per cent, causing some $8.5 trillion in overall losses and eroding nearly four years of output gains.
- The heads of the UN Office on Drugs and Crime, the World Health Organization, the UN High Commissioner for Human Rights, and UNAIDS warned of the heightened vulnerability to COVID-19 of detainees, urging governments to take "all appropriate public health measures" to protect them.
- A new UN report by UN ESCAP noted that the COVID-19 pandemic, due to shutdowns, could help improve the well-being of oceans in the Asia-Pacific region.

14 May

- The Canadian province of Ontario has reported 345 new cases.
- Malaysia has reported 40 new cases bringing the total to 6,819. 70 patients have been discharged, bringing the total number of recoveries to 5,351. Malaysia has also reported one new death, bringing the death toll to 112.
- New Zealand has reported no new cases, with the total remaining at 1,497. Nine people have recovered, bringing the total number of recovered to 1,411.
- Singapore has reported 752 new cases, bringing the total to 26,098.

- Ukraine has reported 422 new cases and 17 new deaths, bringing the total numbers to 16,847 and 456, respectively; a total of 4,143 patients have recovered.
- A total of 126,064 tests for COVID-19 have been conducted in the most recent 24 hour period, the highest number to date.
- Figures compiled by NHS England giving a breakdown of underlying health conditions among COVID-19 hospital fatalities between 31 March and 12 May indicate one in four had diabetes. Other common health conditions were dementia (18%), serious breathing problems (15%), chronic kidney disease (14%), and ischaemic heart disease (10%).
- The Office for National Statistics publishes results of the early phase of a survey programme in England. From swab tests between 27 April and 10 May, they estimate that 148,000 people, or 0.27% of the population, had COVID-19 at any given time during those two weeks (95% confidence interval: 94,000 to 222,000). This implies roughly 10,000 new cases per day. No significant difference is found between broad age groups. Their estimate for people working in healthcare or social care is higher, at 1.33% (confidence interval: 0.39% to 3.28%). The survey does not include people in hospitals or care homes, where rates of infection are likely to be higher still.
- Public Health England approves a blood test developed by Roche Diagnostics that can detect COVID-19 antibodies.
- The Office for Budget Responsibility forecasts the cost to the government of combating the coronavirus pandemic has risen to £123.2bn, with annual borrowing estimated to be

15.2% of the UK economy. This figure is the highest annual borrowing since World War II when it stood at 22.1%.

- The BBC announces plans to resume the filming of EastEnders and Top Gear in June, with the cast and crew practising social distancing and doing their own hair and makeup.
- The UK stages its eighth Clap for Our Carers event at 8 pm.
- Malaysia has reported 40 new cases bringing the total to 6,819. 70 patients have been discharged, bringing the total number of recoveries to 5,351. Malaysia has also reported one new death, bringing the death toll to 112.
- New Zealand has reported no new cases, with the total remaining at 1,497. Nine people have recovered, bringing the total number of recovered to 1,411.
- Singapore has reported 752 new cases, bringing the total to 26,098.
- Ukraine has reported 422 new cases and 17 new deaths, bringing the total numbers to 16,847 and 456, respectively; a total of 4,143 patients have recovered.
- Investigators from the United Nations stated that they deeply regretted Burundi's expulsion of four World Health Organization officials supporting the country's responses to the pandemic.
- The Australian Bureau of Statistics recorded the country's biggest-ever monthly rise in unemployment because of coronavirus lockdown measures. Employment in April dropped by 594,300 to a record of 6.2% unemployment.
- Authorities in the Chinese city of Wuhan begin the planned testing of all 11 million residents of the city after a cluster of new cases was reported at the weekend.

- Japan's Prime Minister Shinzo Abe lifted the state of emergency in most of the country, although it has been retained in Tokyo and Osaka. The Japanese company Takeda Pharmaceutical also announced that it could start a clinical trial by July for a potential COVID-19 treatment based on antibodies collected from a recovered patient's blood.
- New Zealand's Finance Minister Grant Robertson has unveiled a NZ$50 billion fund, equivalent to 17% of the country's GDP, to protect jobs and reduce unemployment to pre-coronavirus levels within two years. The figure is 17 times greater than the sum that the New Zealand government usually allocates to new spending in its budgets.
- Joseph Borrell, the foreign policy chief of the European Union, has called on China to help fight the coronavirus pandemic and called an independent inquiry into the origins of the virus.
- The European Commission halted the delivery of 10 million Chinese face masks after some countries raised concerns over poor quality.
- In Finland, schools have re-opened despite warnings from teachers that it may not be totally safe. Education Minister Li Andersson confirmed the news on April 29.
- France announced travellers coming from Spain must undergo quarantine after Spanish authorities announced a 10-day mandatory quarantine on travellers coming from France. The official said that these measures would be applied to all countries that impose quarantines on arriving French citizens.

- In Italy, the head of the scientific committee, Agostino Miozzo, announced 150,000 citizens in 2,000 urban settlements would undergo testing to help determine the spread of the disease.
- In Poland, it was announced that schools will remain closed until the end of the school year.
- In the United Kingdom, Transport Secretary Grant Shapps announced that a coronavirus test and trace app is being mass-tested on the Isle of Wight.
- The Vatican City has stated that people attending Mass in St. Peter's Basilica will have their temperatures checked upon arrival.
- Investigators from the United Nations stated that they deeply regretted Burundi's expulsion of four World Health Organization officials supporting the country's responses to the pandemic.
- UNAIDS initiated a petition from global leaders requesting that when a successful COVID-19 vaccine is developed, it be available free to all.
- The UN Human Rights High Commissioner warned of potential risks as more countries moved to lift lockdowns to contain COVID-19 spread.
- The UN Secretary-General launched the latest UN policy brief, 'COVID-19 And The Need for Action On Mental Health', urging the international community to do more to protect those facing increasing mental pressures.

15 May

- Government scientific advice says that the R number has increased slightly from between 0.5 and 0.9 to between 0.7 and 1.0, closer to the rate at which infections could start to increase exponentially. The figures are said to be "consistent with" the fall in cases in the community and the rise of cases in care homes but are based on data from three weeks previously, so the effect of easing the lockdown measures is unknown.
- Government scientists and teaching unions hold talks in a bid to safely re-open schools. The British Medical Association voices its support for the unions over their concerns about the safety of resuming classes.
- The place of the worship task force, a body consisting of leading members of faith groups and government representatives, has its inaugural meeting. The group was established in response to Boris Johnson's 10 May address, in which he said religious buildings could re-open by 4 July and aims to examine how this can happen safely.
- Malaysia has reported 36 new cases, bringing the total number of cases to 6,855. There are 1,304 active cases. 88 people have recovered, bringing the total number of recovered to 5,439.
- New Zealand has reported one new case, bringing the total to 1,498 cases (1,148 confirmed and 350 probable). 10 more people have recovered, bringing the total number to 1,421. The new case was linked to the Marist College cluster.
- Singapore has reported 793 new cases, bringing the total to 26,891.

- Ukraine has reported 483 new cases and 20 new deaths, bringing the total numbers to 17,330 and 476, respectively; a total of 4,473 patients have recovered.
- Brazil's health minister Nelson Teich resigned. Teich gave no reason for his choice to resign, stating he had given it "his best."
- The International Monetary Fund has approved a loan of $520 million to assist Jamaica with the country's handling of COVID-19. The Deputy Managing Director of the IMF, Tao Zhang, said that "a sudden stop in tourism and falling remittances" were the primary causes of the need for emergency funds.
- Panama's aviation authority extended its ban on international flights to June 22.
- The US Center for Disease Control has alerted doctors to a "multi-system inflammatory syndrome in children," with current or recent exposure to COVID-19 listed as one of the leading causes.
- In the Australian state of New South Wales, food establishments were allowed to re-open. In the Northern Territory, pubs have re-opened with no restrictions on customer numbers, and the limit on public gatherings and house visits was removed, prompting concerns over a potential rise in infections.
- The Hong Kong economy shrank 8.9% in the first quarter of 2020 amidst the coronavirus pandemic and social unrest in the city.
- In South Korea, the Yonhap news agency has reported that health authorities will disinfect food and drink establishments

in Seoul's nightlife district Itaewon after 17 new infections were linked to the area.

- A study by the World Health Organization has found that coronavirus could potentially infect 231 million people in Africa by the end of 2020. Concerns were raised that the healthcare systems in many African nations could be quickly overrun if there were to be a sudden rise in infections.
- A study by the World Health Organization has found that coronavirus could potentially infect 231 million people in Africa by the end of 2020. Concerns were raised that the healthcare systems in many African nations could be quickly overrun if there were to be a sudden rise in infections.
- The UN refugee agency (UNHCR) reported the first COVID-19 cases in the Cox's Bazar Rohingya refugee camps.
- The UN emergency humanitarian relief agency (OCHA) warned that evacuation centres in the Philippines set up as a response to Typhoon Vongfong were creating the ideal conditions for COVID-19 transmission.
- The UN Office of the High Commissioner for Refugees warned that criminal gangs were exploiting coronavirus lockdowns in Central America.
- UNICEF in the Democratic Republic of the Congo warned coronavirus restrictions affecting vaccinations could result in a resurgence in deadly childhood diseases like "polio, chickenpox, measles, yellow fever, hepatitis B, diphtheria, tetanus, whooping cough, and meningitis."

16 May

- Anne Longfield, the Children's Commissioner for England, urges the government and teaching unions to "stop squabbling and agree a plan" to re-open schools, warning that the closure of schools is negatively affecting disadvantaged children.
- Coronavirus protests involving the gathering of people are held at venues around the UK, including Hyde Park in London and Glasgow Green in Glasgow.
- Malaysia has reported 17 new cases, bringing the total number of cases to 6,782. 73 patients have recovered, bringing the total number to 5,512. Malaysian authorities have also reported one new death, bringing the death toll to 113.
- New Zealand has reported no new cases, with the total number remaining at 1,498. Seven people have recovered, bringing the total number of recoveries to 1,428.
- Singapore has reported 465 new cases, bringing the total to 27,356. Another death was later confirmed, bringing the total to 22.
- Ukraine has reported 528 new cases and 21 new deaths, bringing the total numbers to 17,858 and 497, respectively; a total of 4,473 patients have recovered.
- Air Canada has announced plans to reduce the company's workforce by "50-60 percent", or at least 20,000 employees, as a result of the decline in air travel during the coronavirus pandemic.
- LATAM Airlines has announced it will reduce the company's workforce by 1,400 employees across Latin America, with executive director Roberto Alvo highlighting a large decrease

in business during the pandemic as the primary reason for the decision.

- US President Donald Trump has stated that his government may consider restoring some World Health Organization funds; after all, US contributions were suspended on April 14, potentially in a scenario whereby the US would pay 10% of its former contribution levels.
- The United States House of Representatives passed a $3 trillion bill to reduce the economic and social impacts of the coronavirus on the US. However, Donald Trump's Republican Party stated that the proposal would be "dead on arrival" in the Senate. The bill would provide $1 trillion for regional governments and further payments to families and the unemployed struggling with the crisis.
- The president of the Australian Medical Association, Tony Bartone, urged people to be vigilant after the states of New South Wales and Queensland started easing lockdown restrictions earlier in the week.
- In the Chinese city of Wuhan, health authorities claim to have conducted over 100,000 nucleic acid tests on May 15 after beginning a testing campaign across the whole city in response to a cluster of new domestically transmitted cases was reported to authorities.
- President of Kenya Uhuru Kenyatta has ordered the closure of the country's borders with Somalia and Tanzania for the next 30 days.
- The Tanzanian government has lowered the country's 2020 economic growth projection due to the impact of the coronavirus, with Finance Minister Philip Mpango forecasting growth of 4% compared to an earlier projection of 6.9%.

- President of Zimbabwe Emmerson Mnangagwa has extended the country's coronavirus lockdown but announced that it would be reviewed every two weeks.
- Austrian Chancellor Sebastian Kurz announced that he had reached an agreement with Switzerland and Liechtenstein to fully allow travel across the borders from June 15, whilst confirming that similar talks were being held with the leaders of eastern European countries.
- Authorities in the Czech Republic have said that gatherings of up to 300 people, including sports events, will be allowed later in the month as the country's coronavirus infection rate remained the lowest in Europe. Health Minister Adam Vojtěch said many businesses will be allowed to re-open on May 25.
- Amazon has stated that it aims to begin re-opening its facilities in France on May 19.
- The European Broadcasting Union, organisers of the Eurovision Song Contest, have revealed that an alternative, non-competitive show entitled Eurovision: Europe Shine A Light will be broadcast on May 16. The 2020 edition of the contest was cancelled due to coronavirus.
- Prime Minister of Georgia Giorgi Gakharia will end the state of emergency declared in response to the coronavirus pandemic on May 22.
- In Germany, preliminary data showed their economy had suffered the steepest three-month contraction since the 2008 financial crisis.
- Irish Taoiseach Leo Varadkar has confirmed that the country will introduce a mandatory 14-day quarantine period for

international travellers, although travellers from the British territory of Northern Ireland will be exempt.

- The Portuguese National Institute for Statistics has revealed that Portugal's economy contracted by 3.9% in the first quarter and estimated that the country's GDP shrank by 2.4%.
- In Slovenia, the government has announced an end to the country's coronavirus epidemic. People entering Slovenia from the European Union will no longer have to enter a mandatory seven-day quarantine, although a 14-day quarantine remains in place for arrivals from non-EU countries. The government confirmed that the public will still be expected to keep to "basic rules" to prevent the spread of the virus.
- In the United Kingdom, authorities have approved the manufacture of COVID-19 antibody tests by Abbott Laboratories shortly after giving approval to Swiss company Roche Holding AG.
- President of Kenya Uhuru Kenyatta has ordered the closure of the country's borders with Somalia and Tanzania for the next 30 days.
- The Tanzanian government has lowered the country's 2020 economic growth projection due to the impact of the coronavirus, with Finance Minister Philip Mpango forecasting growth of 4% compared to an earlier projection of 6.9%.
- President of Zimbabwe Emmerson Mnangagwa has extended the country's coronavirus lockdown but announced that it would be reviewed every two weeks.
- The Austrian Government will re-open the country's borders with the Czech Republic, Slovakia, and Hungary from June

15, although restrictions will remain in place for travel to Italy.

- The German Bundesliga resumed after a two-month break during the country's coronavirus lockdown. Finance Minister Olaf Scholz is reportedly preparing an economic stimulus package worth 57 billion euros in response to decreased tax incomes for local municipalities. A number of anti-lockdown protests have occurred across Germany, including a demonstration in Stuttgart with more than 5,000 attendees.
- Prime Minister of Hungary Viktor Orban has announced that lockdown restrictions will be eased in Budapest from May 18, announcing via Facebook that the city will move to the "second phase of defense."
- In Italy, the government will loosen coronavirus travel restrictions, which will see people allowed to move more freely within their home region from May 18, as well as allowing inter-regional journeys from June 3. International travel will also resume from June 3, albeit with strict social distancing rules remaining in place.
- In the United Kingdom, London's Metropolitan Police arrested nineteen people breaking social distancing rules whilst protesting about the government's response to the pandemic in Hyde Park.
- Cambodia will not ease coronavirus lockdown restrictions, despite all infected patients recovering from the virus.
- Reports suggest that hospitals in India's most populous city, Mumbai, are close to collapse as the country deals with the coronavirus.

17 May

- In an article for The Mail on Sunday, Boris Johnson acknowledges frustrations with the government's "stay alert" message for England. Still, he urges the public to be patient as the lockdown measures are eased.
- The number of recorded deaths rose by 170 to 34,636. The daily increase is the lowest since the day after the lockdown restrictions were introduced.
- At the Downing Street daily briefing, Business Secretary Alok Sharma announces a further £84m of funding to help mass-produce a COVID-19 vaccine being trialled by the University of Oxford, and that should be available by September. He also tells the briefing that Oxford has secured an agreement with pharmaceutical company AstraZeneca to manufacture the vaccine and distributed it to the UK first.
- Malaysia has reported 22 new cases, bringing the total number to 6,894. There are 1,210 active cases, while 59 have recovered, bringing the total number of recoveries to 5,571.
- New Zealand has reported one new case, bringing the total number of confirmed and probable cases to 1,499. There remain 45 active cases. Five more people have recovered, bringing the total number of recoveries to 1,433. The latest confirmed case is a Canterbury toddler linked to the Rosewood cluster in Christchurch.
- Singapore has reported 682 new cases, bringing the total to 28,038.

- Ukraine has reported 433 new cases and 17 new deaths, bringing the total numbers to 18,291 and 514, respectively; a total of 5,116 patients have recovered.
- In the Australian state of New South Wales, churches held their first Sunday services since coronavirus lockdown restrictions were imposed in the country, albeit with a heavily reduced capacity.
- Government officials from South Korea and China are reportedly consulting Japan's government in the hope of easing border restrictions between the countries to assist in the recovery of the business.
- Authorities in Sudan announced that all airports in the country will remain closed until May 31.
- India's coronavirus lockdown was extended to May 31.
- A spokeswoman for Indonesia's Ministry of Finance stated that the government is preparing an economic stimulus package of $8.6 billion to support businesses through the pandemic.
- The Sri Lankan government reintroduced a 24-hour curfew for the weekend.
- In Iran, all cities will allow Eid al-Fitr prayers to be held outside after mosques were closed during the Islamic Holy Month of Ramadan due to coronavirus.
- Qatar introduced legislation making the wearing of face masks mandatory in the country, with fines of over $50,000 and three years' jail sentence if caught breaking the rules.
- Reactions and measures in Europe

18 May

- England Rail operators begin running more train services, while security guards trained in crowd control are placed on duty at some major railway stations.
- Jury trials resume at a handful of courts in England and Wales, having been suspended since the beginning of the lockdown restrictions.
- The UK adds loss of smell and loss of taste to the list of COVID-19 symptoms that people should look out for.
- Health Secretary Matt Hancock announces that anyone in the UK over the age of five with symptoms can now be tested for COVID-19.
- Matt Hancock also confirms that 21,000 contact tracers have been recruited across the UK and are ready to begin work.
- Foreign Secretary Dominic Raab tells the Downing Street daily briefing that it is “not sustainable” to keep the lockdown in place “permanently” but that the Government is monitoring the changes it makes.
- Malaysia has reported 47 new cases, bringing the total number of cases to 6,941. 44 have been discharged from the hospital, bringing the total number of recoveries to 5,615. There are 1,213 active cases, with 13 in intensive care and six on ventilator support.
- New Zealand has reported no new cases, recoveries, or deaths; the total number of probable and confirmed cases remains 1,499, recovered cases 1,433, and deaths 21. There remain 45 active cases, with two remaining in hospitals.
- Singapore has reported 305 new cases, bringing the total to 28,343.

- Ukraine has reported 325 new cases and 21 new deaths, bringing the total numbers to 18,616 and 535, respectively; a total of 5,276 patients have recovered.
- Addressing the WHO-sponsored World Health Assembly, the UN Secretary-General warned that a “massive” multilateral effort was needed to tackle the COVID-19 pandemic, as WHO Director-General Tedros Adhanom Ghebreyesus insisted that “the majority of the world’s population remains susceptible to this virus.” On International Museum Day, UNESCO revealed that nearly 90 percent of cultural institutions have had to close, while almost 13 percent were seriously threatened with never re-opening. UN Special Rapporteur on the Rights of Indigenous Peoples, José Francisco Cali Tzay, issued a statement expressing serious concern over the devastating impact of COVID-19 on Indigenous peoples beyond the simple health threat.

19 May

- Figures from the Office for National Statistics show the number of people claiming Jobseeker's Allowance increased by 856,500 in April, to 2.1 million. In response to this, Chancellor Rishi Sunak says that it will take time for the UK economy to recover, and it is "not obvious there will be an immediate bounceback."
- As figures show there have been 11,600 deaths in care homes as a result of COVID-19, Professor Martin Green, chair of Care England, criticises the government for the way it handled the outbreak in care homes and tells MPs they should have been prioritised from the start.

- Security researchers identify major security issues with the NHS COVID-19 tracing app being piloted on the Isle of Wight and call for new legislation to prevent officials from using the data collected for purposes other than identifying those at risk from the virus.
- Captain Tom Moore, who raised £32m for NHS charities, is to be knighted for his fundraising efforts following a special nomination from Boris Johnson.
- China has reported 6 new cases, including one in Wuhan.
- Malaysia has reported 37 new cases, bringing the total number to 6,978. One more death has been reported, bringing the death toll to 114. 31 have recovered, bringing the total number of recovered to 5,646. There are 1,213 active cases, with 11 in intensive care and six on ventilator support.
- New Zealand has reported four new cases, bringing the total number of confirmed and probable cases to 1,503 (1,153 confirmed and 350 probable cases). Nine people have recovered, bringing the total number to 1,442. There are 40 active cases, down from five the day before.
- Singapore has reported 451 new cases, bringing the total to 28,794.
- Ukraine has reported 260 new cases and 13 new deaths, bringing the total numbers to 18,876 and 548, respectively; a total of 5,632 patients have recovered.
- The World Health Organization concluded the annual World Health Assembly, which adopted a resolution calling for an independent review of the global response to the COVID-19 pandemic, including the WHO's performance.

20 May

- At Prime Minister's Questions, Boris Johnson confirms that a track and trace system will be in place from 1 June.
- The Government faces mounting pressure from councils and teaching unions to reconsider its plans to re-open primary schools from 1 June. Robert Buckland, the Secretary of State for Justice, says the Government is taking all concerns "very seriously."
- Rolls-Royce announce plans to cut 9,000 jobs as a result of the COVID-19 outbreak warns that it could take several years for the airline industry to recover.
- The number of people in hospital with COVID-19 has dropped below 10,000 for the first time since March.
- People with diabetes are being strongly advised to follow government advice after a study by NHS England found the condition was linked to a third of coronavirus deaths between 1 March and 11 May. People with diabetes are not among the people who have been told to shield themselves, but some may be asked to do so if they are deemed to be at high risk because of a combination of health conditions.
- At the Downing Street daily briefing, Secretary of State for Digital, Culture, Media, and Sports Oliver Dowden announces the establishment of a task force that will look at how sporting and art events can resume safely. The task force will include former women's footballer Alex Scott and television executive Michael Grade.
- Dowden announces that £150m from dormant bank accounts will be used to help charities and social enterprises.

- The 2020 Queen's Birthday Honours is delayed until autumn in order to recognise the "everyday Covid heroes" who have played a role in supporting and protecting society during the crisis.
- Figures released by Public Health England indicate no new coronavirus cases were reported in London over the 24 hours up to Monday 18 May.
- Malaysia has reported 31 new cases, bringing the total to 7,009. 60 patients have been discharged, bringing the total number of recoveries to 5,706. There are 1,189 active cases in hospitals, with 11 in intensive care and seven on ventilator support.
- New Zealand has reported five new recoveries, bringing the total number of recoveries to 1,447. There are 35 active cases, with one case remaining in hospital. The total number of probable and confirmed cases stands at 1,503, while the death toll remains at 21.
- Singapore has reported 570 new cases, bringing the total to 29,364.
- Ukraine has reported 354 new cases and 16 new deaths, bringing the total numbers to 19,230 and 564, respectively; a total of 5,955 patients have recovered.
- The New Zealand Ministry of Health officially launched a contact tracing app called NZ COVID Tracer, available on App Store and Google Play. It allows users to scan their QR codes at businesses, public buildings, and other organisations to track where they have been for contract tracing purposes.
- At the launch of a UN briefing paper focusing on the impact of COVID-19 across Africa, the UN Secretary-General called

for solidarity to preserve Africa's hard-won progress. At the same time, the UN High Commissioner for Human Rights and the Chairperson of the African Commission on Human and Peoples' Rights issued a joint call for urgent measures to reduce the ripple effects of COVID-19 on Africa's most vulnerable, warning that hoping it would go away would not work.

21 May

- The NHS Confederation warns that time is running out to finalise a test, track and trace strategy to avoid a possible second surge in coronavirus cases.
- Following an agreement between the Government and the Swiss pharmaceutical company Roche, a COVID-19 antibody test is made available through the NHS, with health and care staff to be the first to receive it. The test checks to see if someone has had the virus.
- The Government announces that NHS staff and care workers from overseas will be exempt from the immigration health surcharge that usually applies to non-EU migrants.
- The Office for National Statistics estimates that 137,000 people in England, or 0.25% of the population, had COVID-19 at any given time between 4 May and 17 May (excluding those in hospitals, care homes, or other institutions). This implies around 8,700 new infections per day, compared to the 10,000 estimates made two weeks ago.
- ITV announces that its soap Emmerdale has started a "phased return to filming" with six new episodes being recorded at its studios in Leeds.
- The UK stages its ninth weekly Clap for Our Carers event at 8 pm.

- Malaysia has reported 50 new cases, bringing the total to 7,050. There are 1,149 active cases, ten in intensive care and seven on respirator support. 90 people were discharged, bringing the total number of recoveries to 5,796.
- New Zealand has reported five new recoveries, bringing the total number to 1,452. There are 30 active cases, with one remaining in the hospital. The total number of probable and confirmed cases stands at 1,502, while the death toll remains 21.
- Singapore has reported 448 new cases, bringing the total to 29,812. Another death was later confirmed, bringing the total to 23.
- Ukraine has reported 476 new cases and 15 new deaths, bringing the total numbers to 19,706 and 579, respectively; a total of 6,227 patients have recovered.
- UN Secretary-General António Guterres launches a new UN initiative dubbed Verified to fight COVID-19 misinformation.
- The UN Secretary-General launched Verified, led by the UN's Department of Global Communications, to create a cadre of "digital-first responders" to increase the volume and reach of trusted, accurate information on the COVID-19 crisis.
- UNICEF warned that migrant children forcibly returned from the United States to Mexico and Central America were facing danger and discrimination worsened by the COVID-19 pandemic.
- The World Health Organization (WHO) and UN refugee agency (UNHCR) signed a new pact, an update, and expansion of a 1997 agreement, funded by the COVID-19 Solidarity Response Fund, to better protect approximately 70

million people affected by COVID-19 in low and middle-income countries with vulnerable health systems.

22 May

- The British Government unveils new quarantine rules for travellers to the UK that will require them to self-isolate for fourteen days from 8 June.
- The Scientific Advisory Group for Emergencies published its evidence on the safety and impact of re-opening schools on 1 June. It says the risk to school pupils is "very, very small, but it is not zero," while the risk to teachers is not above average compared to other occupations.
- The Office for National Statistics reports that government borrowing rose to £62bn in April, the highest monthly figure on record, after heavy spending to ease the coronavirus crisis.
- Guernsey announces plans to move to Stage Four of its lockdown restrictions from 30 May, six weeks earlier than originally planned. This will allow restaurants and cafes, hairdressers and beauticians, cinemas, gyms, and sports venues to re-open. The announcement comes after the island had 22 consecutive days with no new COVID-19 cases. Schools on the island will also re-open for all students on 8 June.
- Annemarie Plas, credited as starting the weekly Clap for Our Carers, suggests it should end after its tenth week as the public has shown their appreciation. Instead, it should become an annual celebration of frontline workers.
- Malaysia has reported 78 new cases, bringing the total number to 7,137. There are 1,163 active cases, with nine in intensive care and five on ventilator support. 63 have

recovered, bringing the total number of recoveries to 5,859. Malaysia also reported one new death, bringing the death toll to 115.

- New Zealand has reported one new case, bringing the total number of probable and confirmed cases to 1,504. Three people have recovered, bringing the total number of recoveries to 1,455. There are 28 active cases, with one in the hospital.
- Singapore has reported 614 new cases, bringing the total to 30,426.
- Ukraine has reported 442 new cases and 9 new deaths, bringing the total numbers to 20,148 and 588, respectively; a total of 6,585 patients have recovered.
- US President Donald Trump designated churches, mosques, and synagogues as "essential services" and called upon state governors to allow them to re-open, criticizing the decision by some state governors to allow liquor stores and abortion clinics to re-open but not churches. State and local officials have the authority to designate essential services and issue stay-at-home orders, however.
- The UN Office for the Coordination of Humanitarian Affairs warned that war-torn Yemen's health system had 'in effect, collapsed" in the face of a widening COVID-19 outbreak.
- On International Day for Biological Diversity, the UN Secretary-General called for the world to build back better and preserve biodiversity after the COVID-19 pandemic.
- . The Director-General of the World Health Organization reiterated that the COVID-19 pandemic disrupted access to routine immunization services worldwide, increasing the risk

of potentially lethal diseases like diphtheria, measles, and pneumonia.

- Malaysian Prime Minister Muhyiddin Yassin entered into a 14-day quarantine after an officer attending a post-Cabinet meeting on 21 May tested positive for COVID-19.

23 May

- The French Government announces that travellers to France from the UK will have to quarantine for 14 days from 8 June.
- The death of a 12-year-old child is reported.
- Dominic Cummings, Boris Johnson's chief political adviser, comes under mounting pressure to resign after a joint investigation by the Daily Mirror, and The Guardian reported that he travelled 260 miles from London to Durham to self-isolate during the lockdown. In response to the story, Downing Street says that Cummings travelled to the northeast to be near relatives who could look after his young son if he became ill himself.
- Transport Secretary Grant Shapps announces £283m of investment in buses and light rail services in order to help improve safety but warns capacity will be at a fifth of pre-lockdown levels because of social distancing measures. Extra Martials at stations from 1 June are also announced and permission for ten rail re-opening projects to proceed to make business cases under the "reversing the Beeching cuts" initiative.
- Malaysia has reported 48 new cases, bringing the total to 7,185. There have been 1,158 active cases, with nine in intensive care and five on ventilator support. 53 have been discharged, bringing the total number of recoveries to 5,912. The death toll stands at 115.

- New Zealand has reported no new cases, deaths, or recoveries. The total number of confirmed and probable cases stands at 1,504; the death toll at 21; and the number of recoveries at 1,455.
- Singapore has reported 642 new cases, bringing the total to 31,068.
- Ukraine has reported 432 new cases and 17 new deaths, bringing the total numbers to 20,580 and 605, respectively; a total of 6,929 patients have recovered.
- US car Rental Company Hertz files for Chapter 11 bankruptcy protection as a result of the economic effects of the COVID-19 pandemic. The company had already laid off 10,000 employees and is facing US$14 billion in debts.

24 May

- After The Observer and the Sunday Mirror print allegations that Dominic Cummings made a second trip to the northeast during the lockdown, Boris Johnson gives his chief aide his backing at the Downing Street daily briefing, saying that Cummings had "no alternative" but to travel for childcare "when both he and his wife were about to be incapacitated by coronavirus" and has "acted responsibly, legally and with integrity." Johnson describes some of the claims as "palpably false."
- Johnson also confirms plans (outlined on 10 May) for the phased re-opening of schools in England from 1 June: from that date, they will re-open for early years pupils, Reception, Year 1 and Year 6. For the first time, he states that from 15 June, a quarter of Year 10 and Year 12 students will be allowed "some contact" to help prepare for exams.

- Brazil has reported a total of over 363,000 cases and nearly 23,000 deaths.
- Malaysia has reported 60 new cases, bringing the total to 7,245. There are 1,185 active cases, with nine in intensive care and four on ventilator support. 33 have been discharged, bringing the total number of recoveries to 5,945. The death toll remains at 115.
- New Zealand has reported one new recovery, bringing the total recoveries to 1,456 and leaving 27 active cases. The total number of confirmed and probable cases remains at 1,154, and the death toll at 21.
- Singapore has reported 548 new cases, bringing the total to 31,616.
- Ukraine has reported 406 new cases and 12 new deaths, bringing the total numbers to 20,986 and 617, respectively; a total of 7,108 patients have recovered.

25 May

- Dominic Cummings says, "I don't regret what I did," as he gives a detailed explanation of his actions during lockdown at a press conference in the Downing Street Rose Garden.
- Education Secretary Gavin Williamson warns the virus "could be with us for a year or more," and children cannot stay off school for "months and months."
- Malaysia has reported 172 new cases, bringing the total number of cases to 7,417. There are 1,410 active cases. 34 were discharged, bringing the total number of recoveries to 5,979. The death toll remains at 115.
- New Zealand has reported no new cases, recoveries, and deaths, which remain at 1,504 (1,154 confirmed and 350

probable), 1,456, and 21, respectively. There are 27 active cases.

- The Philippines has reported 284 new cases, bringing the total to 14,319. The Philippines also reported that 74 have recovered, bringing the total to 3,323. There were five new deaths, bringing the death toll to 873.
- Singapore has reported 344 new cases, bringing the total to 31,960.
- Ukraine has reported 259 new cases and 6 new deaths, bringing the total numbers to 21,245 and 623, respectively; a total of 7,108 patients have recovered.
- New Zealand Prime Minister Jacinda Ardern announced that the limit on social gatherings like religious services, weddings, and funerals would be raised to 100 at 12 pm on 29 May 2020. She also announced that Cabinet would make a decision on moving into Alert level 1 on 8 June, with 22 June set as the tentative date for moving into alert level 1. That same day, MediaWorks CEO Michael Anderson announced that the company would be eliminating 130 jobs in its sales, out-of-home, and radio divisions due to the economic effects of the coronavirus pandemic.

26 May

- For the first day since 18 March, no new COVID deaths have been reported in Northern Ireland. Robin Swann, the Northern Ireland Health Minister, describes it as "a clear sign of progress."
- Death registration figures for the week ending 15 May show the lowest number of COVID-19 deaths since the beginning of April.

- Remdesivir, a drug that can speed up the recovery time of patients with COVID-19, is made available through the NHS.
- Douglas Ross resigns as a junior minister with the Scotland Office over the UK government's defense of Dominic Cummings. At the same time, at least 35 Conservative MPs call for Cummings to be removed from his post.
- Tate Britain announces that the annual Turner Prize will not be awarded in 2020 because of the upheaval created by the COVID outbreak.
- Malaysia has reported 187 new cases (10 imported and 177 local transmissions), bringing the total number to 7,604. Of the 177 local transmissions, 173 involved foreigners detained at immigration detention centres. 62 have been discharged, bringing the total number of recoveries to 6,041. There are 1,448 active cases in Malaysia, with eight in intensive care and five on ventilator support.
- New Zealand has reported five new recoveries, bringing the total number of recovered to 1,461. There are 22 active cases, with the total number confirmed and probable cases remaining 1,504. The death toll has remained at 21.
- Singapore has reported 383 new cases, bringing the total to 32,343.
- Ukraine has reported 339 new cases and 21 new deaths, bringing the total numbers to 21,584 and 644, respectively; a total of 7,575 patients have recovered.
- The George Floyd protests begin in Minneapolis. Largely via social media, they later spread throughout the country and around the world. Health experts and public officials have expressed concerns that these mass gatherings may cause an exacerbated spread of the virus since May 31st or earlier.

27 May

- Boris Johnson states that a test and trace system will be operational in England from the following day.
- Johnson appears before the House of Commons Liaison Committee, where he rules out holding an inquiry into the actions of Dominic Cummings.
- Figures from HM Treasury indicate the Coronavirus Job Retention Scheme for furloughed workers in the UK now covers 8.4 million people, an increase from 8 million a week earlier.
- Malaysia has reported 15 new cases (the lowest figure since the movement control order began on 18 March), bringing the total to 7,619. 42 have been discharged, bringing the total number of recoveries to 6,083. There are 1,421 active cases, with six in intensive care and four on ventilator support. The death toll remains at 115.
- New Zealand has reported one new recovery, bringing the total number of recovered to 1,462. There are 21 active cases, with the total number of confirmed and probable cases remaining 1,504. The death toll still stands at 21.
- Singapore has reported 533 new cases, bringing the total to 32,876.
- Ukraine has reported 321 new cases and 14 new deaths, bringing the total numbers to 21,905 and 658, respectively; a total of 7,995 patients have recovered.
- The United States has reported 100,000 deaths as a result of the COVID-19 pandemic, with 29,000 recorded in New York State.

- The ILO warned in a new report that more than one in six young people had stopped working since the beginning of the pandemic, creating a 'lockdown generation.'
- The WHO Foundation, an independent body, was launched to help fund the WHO as "an integral part of the UN agency's resource mobilization strategy to broaden its donor base."

28 May

- Contact tracing systems go live in England and Scotland – NHS Test and Trace in England, and Test and Protect in Scotland. However, Dido Harding tells MPs the system in England will not be "fully operational at a local level" until the end of June.
- The weekly household survey by the Office for National Statistics reports that around 133,000 people in England had COVID-19 at any given time during 11–24 May. It estimates the rate of new infections to be around 54,000 per week. Both numbers are similar to the previous estimates, indicating that the number of infections is "relatively stable."
- A meeting of the four national Chief Medical Officers decides that the alert level should remain at 4, although Boris Johnson had said the previous day that he hoped it would come down to 3.
- Durham Police say that Dominic Cummings may have made a "minor breach" of lockdown rules during his visit to Barnard Castle, but no offense was committed.
- EasyJet announces plans to cut 4,500 jobs because of the effects of the COVID-19 outbreak on business.
- The tenth and final Clap for Our Carers event is staged at 8 pm.

- Malaysia has reported ten new cases, bringing the total number to 7,629. 86 patients have been discharged, bringing the total number of recoveries to 6,169. There are 1,345 active cases, with eight in intensive care and four on ventilator support. The death toll remains at 115.
- New Zealand has reported 12 new recoveries, bringing the total number of recovered to 1,474. . 8 active cases remain after a death was reported to be linked to the St Margaret's rest home cluster in Auckland, bringing the death toll to 22. The total number of cases remains at 1,504 (1,154 confirmed and 350 probable).
- Russia has reported 174 deaths, bringing the death toll to 4,142. Russia has also reported 8,371 new cases, bringing the total to 379,051.
- Singapore has reported 373 new cases, bringing the total to 33,249.
- Ukraine has reported 477 new cases and 11 new deaths, bringing the total numbers to 22,382 and 669, respectively; a total of 8,439 patients have recovered.
- The WFP released projections showing that approximately 14 million people in Latin America and the Caribbean could experience extreme food insecurity in 2020 due to the COVID-19 pandemic.
- The UN Secretary-General called for greater "unite and solidarity" at a high-level funding meeting as he warned of 60 million pushed into extreme poverty; coming famines of “historic proportions”; approximately 1.6 billion people unemployed; and a 'Great Depression'-like loss of $8.5 trillion in global output.

- UN agencies and global partners announced they were seeking $2.41 billion to fight COVID-19 spread in Yemen and support millions affected in the "world's worst humanitarian crisis."
- The Malaysian Ministry of National Unity announced that a total of 174 non-Muslim houses of worship have been allowed to resume operations from 10 June according to the "Standard Operating Procedure for Houses of Worship in Green Zones." Marriages at temples, churches, and religious associations have been postponed until 31 July 2020.

29 May

- Chancellor Rishi Sunak announces that the Coronavirus Job Retention Scheme will end at the end of October. Before then, employers must pay National Insurance and pension contributions from August, then 10% of pay from September, increasing to 20% in October. . In August, self-employed people whose work has been affected by the outbreak will receive a "second and final" government grant.
- Malaysia has reported 103 new cases, bringing the total to 7,732. 66 patients have been discharged, bringing the total number of recoveries to 6,235. There are 1,382 active cases, with eight in intensive care and two on ventilator support.
- New Zealand has reported seven new recoveries, bringing the total number of recoveries to 1,481. There is one active case, with the total number of cases being 1,504 (1,154 confirmed and 350 probable). The death toll remains at 22.
- Singapore has reported 611 new cases, bringing the total to 33,860.

- Ukraine has reported 429 new cases and 10 new deaths, bringing the total numbers to 22,811 and 679, respectively; a total of 8,934 patients have recovered.
- A partial easing of the stay-at-home order in Illinois, except for Chicago, was scheduled to occur.
- Thirty countries and multiple international partners signed up to support the WHO-backed COVID-19 Technology Access Pool (C-TAP), a “one-stop-shop” for sharing data, intellectual property, and scientific knowledge to counter the disease.
- Reactions and measures in Africa.

30 May

- Some government scientific advisers warn of the risk associated with lifting lockdown restrictions in England too early, citing the still high number of cases and deaths. In response, the government says it is following the data and evidence when making its decisions about the restrictions. Professor Jonathan Van-Tam tells the Downing Street briefing that Britain is "dangerous moment" and people must be "sensible and proportionate."
- At the Downing Street daily briefing, Culture Secretary Oliver Dowden announces that competitive sport will be allowed in England behind closed doors from 1 June, with individual sporting bodies left to decide when to restart. Horse racing will be one of the first sporting activities to resume.
- Conservative MPs urge Boris Johnson to revise the 2 metre social distancing rule to 1.5 metres amid concerns for the hospitality industry.
- Malaysia has reported 30 new cases, bringing the total number to 7,762. 95 patients have been discharged, bringing

the total number of recovered to 6,330. There are 1,137 active cases, with nine patients in intensive care and two on ventilator support. The death toll remains at 115.

- New Zealand has reported no new cases, recoveries, or deaths, with the total number remaining 1,504, 1,481, and 22, respectively. There remains only one active case.
- Singapore has reported 506 new cases, bringing the total to 34,366.
- Ukraine has reported 393 new cases and 17 new deaths, bringing the total numbers to 23,204 and 696, respectively; a total of 9,311 patients have recovered.

31 May

- The UK exceeds its target to increase testing capacity to 200,000 tests a day by the end of May, with 205,634 available for 30 May.
- Malaysia has reported 57 new cases (10 imported and 47 local transmissions), bringing the total to 7,819 cases. 23 have been discharged, bringing the total number of recovered to 6,353. There are 1,351 active cases, with nine in intensive care and two on ventilator support.
- New Zealand has reported no new cases, recoveries, or deaths, with the total number remaining 1,504, 1,481, and 22, respectively. There remains only one active case.
- Singapore has reported 518 new cases, bringing the total to 34,884. Tests on all nursing homes found almost all residents and staff healthy except for five cases detected earlier.

- Ukraine has reported 468 new cases and 12 new deaths, bringing the total numbers to 23,672 and 708, respectively; a total of 9,538 patients have recovered.
- The stay-at-home orders in Alameda County, California; Contra Costa County, California; Marin County, California; San Mateo County, California; Santa Clara County, California; Berkeley, California; and San Francisco, California are scheduled to end.

Pandemic Chronology June 2020

1 June

- Malaysia has reported 38 new cases, bringing the total to 7,857. There are 1,338 active cases, with eight in intensive care and two on ventilator support. 51 patients have been discharged, bringing the number of recovered to 6,404. The death toll remains at 115.
- New Zealand has reported no new cases, recoveries, and deaths, which remain at 1,504 (1,154 confirmed and 350 probable), 1,481, and 22, respectively. There remains one active case.
- Singapore has reported 408 new cases, bringing the total to 35,292. Another death was later confirmed, bringing the total to 24.
- Ukraine has reported 340 new cases and 10 new deaths, bringing the total numbers to 24,012 and 718 respectively; a total of 9,690 patients have recovered.
- The Health Protection (Coronavirus, Restrictions) (England) (Amendment No. 3) Regulations 2020 (SI 558) come into effect, again without prior parliamentary scrutiny. Car and caravan showrooms, outdoor sports amenities, and outdoor non-food markets may re-open. The prohibitions on leaving home are replaced by a prohibition on staying overnight away from home, with specific exceptions. Gatherings of people from more than one household are limited to six people outdoors and are prohibited entirely indoors, with exceptions including education. There are further exemptions for elite athletes.

- ITV announces plans to resume filming of its soap Coronation Street from 9 June following an eleven-week break. ITV has aired three episodes a week since March, and the new filming schedule will allow that number of airings to continue.
- The World Health Organization (WHO) published research finding that the fight against COVID-19 had severely disrupted services to prevent and treat non-communicable diseases like cancer, diabetes, and hypertension, which kill over 40 million people each year.
- Dr. Michael Ryan, WHO Executive Director, highlighted that Central and South America were now 'intense zones' for COVID-19 transmission.
- The World Tourism Organization (UNWTO) published research noting that countries were cautiously starting to ease travel restrictions.
- In New Zealand, Microbiologist and health adviser Dr. Siouxsie Wiles, Deputy Prime Minister Winston Peters, and ACT Party leader David Seymour have criticized protesters who attended protests in several centers, including Auckland and Wellington, for flouting social distancing restrictions. Dr. Wiles called for people who attended the BLM marches and gatherings to self-isolate for 14 days. Peters and Seymour also called for the New Zealand Government to move from alert level 2 to level 1.

2 June

- Malaysia has reported 20 new cases (15 imported and five locally transmitted), bringing the total number to 7,877. 66 patients have recovered, bringing the total number to 6,470. There are 1,292 active cases, six in intensive care and two on ventilator support. The death toll has remained at 115.
- New Zealand has reported no new cases, recoveries, and deaths, which remain at 1,504 (1,154 confirmed and 350 probable), 1,481, and 22, respectively. There remains one active case. Director-General of Health Ashley Bloomfield confirmed that 654 tests were completed on Monday, bringing the total number of tests to 282,263.
- Singapore has reported 544 new cases, bringing the total to 35,836.
- Ukraine has reported 328 new cases and 9 new deaths, bringing the total numbers to 24,340 and 727, respectively; a total of 10,078 patients have recovered.
- Figures from the Office for National Statistics show the number of COVID-19 deaths at their lowest since March, with 2,872 death certificates mentioning the condition during the week up to 22 May.
- The Guardian has calculated the UK death toll from COVID-19 is 50,032. Meanwhile, Reuters gives the figure as 49,646.
- David Norgrove, chair of the UK Statistics Authority, rebukes Matt Hancock in an escalation of his 11 May criticism of the government's handling of testing data, saying the figures are "still far from complete and comprehensible" and appear to be aimed at showing "the largest possible number of tests, even at the expense of understanding."

- MPs vote to end the practice of voting from home, but some politicians criticise the move for excluding those unable to attend Parliament due to age or health reasons. In response, Jacob Rees-Mogg, the Leader of the House, says he will schedule a motion for the following day that will enable them to question the government but not to vote.
- Water companies urge people to conserve water during the lockdown restrictions by not using sprinklers and hosepipes or filling paddling pools. The advice follows a record dry spring coupled with more people spending time at home.
- The Royal Shakespeare Company announces it has called off performances planned for the summer, autumn and winter because of the COVID-19 outbreak.
- The England and Wales Cricket Board confirms England will play three test matches against the West Indies starting on 8 July.
- The UK government is to scale back its daily Downing Street briefings to weekdays only, citing low viewing figures at weekends. Boris Johnson will also commit to leading one briefing per week.
- Singapore Airlines has announced that it will resume passenger flights to the New Zealand cities of Auckland and Christchurch on a weekly basis. In addition, the Singaporean national carrier announced that it will be resuming flights to the Australian cities of Adelaide, Melbourne, and Brisbane while establishing new routes to Sydney between 8 June and 31 July.
- The President of the General Assembly, Tijani Muhammad-Bande, called for UN Member States to place human rights

at the heart of their ongoing response to COVID-19 and ensure that everyone can enjoy "justice and peace."

- At a UN ECOSOC Financing for Development Forum, exploring financing options to address the pandemic and mobilize the resources needed for a proactive recovery, Deputy Secretary-General Amina J. Mohammed informed delegates that 'unprecedented' financing was needed to halt a recession of 'unparalleled proportions':
- The UN High Commissioner for Human Rights called for urgent action to address "the major disproportionate impact" of COVID-19 on racial and ethnic minorities, including people of African descent.
- At a virtual pledging conference for Yemen, where community transmission of the coronavirus was likely underway, the UN Secretary-General warned that the country, whose health system had collapsed, was facing a massive humanitarian crisis and was "hanging on by a thread."
- Gilbert F. Houngbo, President of the International Fund for Agricultural Development, warned that due to the coronavirus, cross-border remittances will fall by 20 percent, or $110 billion, to $445 billion, potentially causing tens of millions to fall below the poverty line and undermining progress towards fulfilling the 2030 Agenda for Sustainable Development.

3 June

- Malaysia has reported 93 new cases, bringing the total number to 7,970. There are 1,324 active cases, six in intensive care and two on ventilator support. 61 patients have recovered, bringing the total number of recovered to 6,531. The death toll remains at 115.
- New Zealand has reported no new cases, recoveries, and deaths, which remain at 1,504 (1,154 confirmed and 350 probable), 1,481, and 22, respectively. There remains one active case.
- Singapore has reported 569 new cases, bringing the total to 36,405.
- Ukraine has reported 483 new cases and 8 new deaths, bringing the total numbers to 24,823 and 735, respectively; a total of 10,440 patients have recovered.
- Home Secretary Priti Patel confirms plans to introduce a 14-day quarantine for new arrivals into the UK. Those who break the quarantine conditions in England will face fines of £1,000 and potential prosecution.
- Business Secretary Alok Sharma is tested for COVID-19 and self-isolates at home after looking visibly ill during a House of Commons debate. He subsequently tests negative for the virus.
- As the UK begins a period of wetter weather, Boris Johnson urges people not to move gatherings indoors if it rains.
- The UN Secretary-General, António Guterres, launched the latest UN policy briefing on the pandemic, which reminds countries of their obligation to protect people on the move, now more than 70 million globally, according to data from the UN refugee agency, UNHCR, expressing optimism that the

COVID-19 crisis would lead to a rethinking of how the world supports refugees, migrants, and internally displaced people.

- UN High Commissioner for Human Rights Michelle Bachelet urged Asian-Pacific countries to honour the right to freedom of expression, following an alarming clampdown on freedom of expression during the COVID-19 crisis.
- On World Bicycle Day, the World Health Organization highlighted the potential for bicycles to transform the way the world moves around and create a healthier, more sustainable future after the pandemic.
- The Secretary-General appealed for greater unity and solidarity to defeat COVID-19 and build a better world in its wake opening remarks to an extraordinary inter-sessional summit of the 79-member Organization of African, Caribbean, and the Pacific States.
- New Zealand Prime Minister Jacinda Ardern announced that the Government would consider moving into an Alert level 1 lockdown on 8 June. She clarified that Alert level 1 would involve the elimination of social distancing restrictions on shops, restaurants, public transportation, and public gatherings, including religious services, funerals, weddings, and community sports events. However, event organisers would have to ensure contact tracing.
- On 3 June, Malaysian Education Minister Dr. Mohd Radzi Md Jidin announced that the Government would be distributing guidelines to teachers on 4 June as part of plans to re-open the education sector.

4 June

- Malaysia has reported 277 new cases, bringing the total to 8,247. There are 1,573 active cases, six in intensive care and two on ventilator support. 28 patients have recovered, bringing the total number of recovered to 6,559.
- New Zealand has reported no new cases, recoveries, and deaths, which remain at 1,504 (1,154 confirmed and 350 probable), 1,481, and 22, respectively. There remains one active case.
- Singapore has reported 517 new cases, bringing the total to 36,922.
- Ukraine has reported record 588 new cases as well as 12 new deaths, bringing the total numbers to 25,411 and 747, respectively; a total of 11,042 patients have recovered.
- Debenhams announces plans to re-open three stores in Northern Ireland from 8 June, followed by 50 in England a week later.
- Research by King's College London has suggested that half the UK population has struggled with sleep during the lockdown.

5 June

- Malaysia has reported 19 new cases, bringing the total number of cases to 8,266. 51 patients have recovered, bringing the total number of recoveries to 6,610. There are 1,540 active cases, with six in intensive care and one on ventilator support. Malaysia has reported one new death, bringing the total to 116.
- New Zealand has reported no new cases, recoveries, and deaths, which remain at 1,504 (1,154 confirmed and 350

probable), 1,481, and 22, respectively. There remains one active case.

- Singapore has reported 261 new cases, bringing the total to 37,183.
- Ukraine has reported 553 new cases and 15 new deaths, bringing the total numbers to 25,964 and 762, respectively; a total of 11,372 patients have recovered.
- The number of recorded deaths passes 40,000 after rising by 357 to 40,261.
- The British Medical Association urges the UK government to extend the rules regarding the wearing of face-covering to all situations where social distancing is not possible.
- Sir Patrick Vallance, the UK's Government Chief Scientific Adviser, says the R number is between 0.7 and 0.9 but could be as high as 1 in some areas of England. His comments come after figures from the Office for National Statistics suggest the reproductive rate is between 0.7 and 1 for England.
- The weekly household survey by the Office for National Statistics reports that around 53,000 people (95% confidence: 25,000 to 99,000) in England had COVID-19 at any given time during 17–30 May. It estimates the rate of new infections to be around 39,000 per week, down from 54,000 the previous week. Their estimates are based on small numbers: 21 positive results from just under 20,000 swab tests.
- The UK government's ban on tenant evictions in England and Wales is extended by two months to 23 August.

- Health Secretary Matt Hancock urges people not to breach lockdown rules by attending protests planned for the forthcoming weekend. Several are planned by the organisation Black Lives Matter following the killing of George Floyd in the United States.
- The World Health Organization, in updated guidance, stated that governments in areas with widespread COVID-19 transmission should encourage the use of non-medical masks on public transport, in shops, and other confined locations.
- The Under-Secretary-General for Peace Operations warned that in the Sahel African subregion, terrorist groups were exploiting the pandemic as they increased attacks on national and international peacekeeping forces.
- Governor of California Gavin Newsom announced that the state's entertainment industry can resume film, television, and music production on 12 June following a three and a half month shutdown. However, studios and labor unions will have to abide by new safety protocols issued by the California Department of Public Health to protect workers from the spread of COVID-19.

6 June

- Malaysia has reported 37 new cases, bringing the total number of cases to 8,303. There are 1,551 cases, with five in intensive care. 25 patients have recovered, bringing the total number of recovered to 6,635. The country has reported one new death, bringing the death toll to 117.
- New Zealand has reported no new cases, recoveries, and deaths, which remain at 1,504 (1,154 confirmed and 350

probable), 1,481, and 22, respectively. There remains one active case.

- Singapore has reported 344 new cases, bringing the total to 37,527. Another death was later confirmed, bringing the total to 25.
- Ukraine has reported 550 new cases and 15 new deaths, bringing the total numbers to 26,514 and 777, respectively; a total of 11,812 patients have recovered.
- Anti-racism demonstrations are held in cities across the UK; attendees are reported to be in the thousands.
- Robert Jenrick announces that places of worship will be allowed to open for individual prayer on 15 June.
- The Malaysian Director-General of Health Noor Hisham Abdullah has advised Malaysians to wear face masks in response to a World Health Organization directive encouraging people to wear face masks. He also confirmed that the country's movement control order would remain in force since the country is still being monitored under the Prevention and Control of Infectious Diseases Act 1988. Noor Hisham also confirmed that hair and beauty salons could re-open as long as they adhered to social distancing measures.

7 June

- Malaysia has reported 19 new cases, bringing the total to 8,322. There are 1,531 active cases, with five in intensive care. 39 were discharged, bringing the total number of recovered to 6,674.
- New Zealand has reported no new cases, recoveries, and deaths, which remain at 1,504 (1,154 confirmed and 350

probable), 1,481, and 22, respectively. There remains one active case.

- Singapore has reported 383 new cases, bringing the total to 37,910.
- Ukraine has reported 485 new cases and 11 new deaths, bringing the total numbers to 26,999 and 788, respectively; a total of 12,054 patients have recovered.
- No new deaths are recorded for Scotland or Northern Ireland over the most recent 24 hour period; it is the first time Scotland has recorded no new deaths since lockdown began in March.
- Thousands of protesters take part in the second day of anti-racism demonstrations in cities across the UK.
- Professor John Edmunds, one of the scientists advising the UK government, says he wishes the lockdown had been implemented earlier as the delay "cost a lot of lives but adds that data was "really quite poor,"making it "very hard" to do act earlier. Responding to the comments, Health Secretary Matt Hancock says the government "took the right decision at the right time."
- Malaysian Prime Minister Muhyiddin Yassin announced that the country's movement control order would end on 9 June, with the country moving into the Recovery Movement Control Order (RMCO) phase between 10 June and 31 August. Under this arrangement, interstate travel will be allowed except for areas under Enhanced Movement Control Order (EMCO) and domestic tourism, barbers, beauty shops, night markets, bazaars, museums, indoor busking, and fishing, and filming. Schools will re-open in stages.

Large gatherings and sports involving many people will still be disallowed, as well as international travel.

8 June

- Malaysia has reported seven new cases, bringing the total to 8,329. 20 patients have been discharged, bringing the total number of recovered to 6,694. There are 1,518 active cases, with six in intensive care and one on ventilator support. The death toll remains at 117.
- New Zealand's last active case has recovered, meaning that the country has no active cases and bringing the number of recovered to 1,482. The country has reported a total number of 1,504 cases (1,154 confirmed and 350 probable) and 22 deaths.
- Singapore has reported 386 new cases, bringing the total to 38,296.
- Ukraine has reported 463 new cases and 9 new deaths, bringing the total numbers to 27,462 and 797, respectively; a total of 12,195 patients have recovered.
- Rules requiring travellers arriving into the UK to quarantine for 14 days come into force.
- The number of recorded deaths rises by 55 to 40,597, the lowest daily number since lockdown was introduced on 23 March; no deaths are reported in Scotland for a second consecutive day, and there are no new deaths in London hospitals.
- BP announces plans to shed 10,000 jobs amid a global drop in demand for oil.
- The World Bank stated in its latest Global Economic Prospects report. that the COVID-19 pandemic would shrink

the global economy by 5.2 percent in 2020, the deepest recession since World War Two, triggering a dramatic rise in extreme poverty.

- The World Health Organization warned that the COVID-19 pandemic was worsening globally, with more than 136,000 cases recorded on 7 June, the highest ever in a single day.
- New Zealand Prime Minister Jacinda Ardern announced that the country would be entering into Alert level 1 at midnight on 9 June after it was reported that the country's last remaining active case had recovered. Under an Alert level 1 lockdown, social distancing would stop with no restrictions on daily life, business activities, mass gatherings, and public transportation but the country's borders would remain closed to most international travel.
- British Home Secretary Priti Patel has announced that all people entering the United Kingdom will have to provide an address where they can self-isolate for 14 days or face fines of £1,000. Travelers exempt from this ruling include anyone arriving from the Republic of Ireland, the Channel Islands, or the Isle of Man and workers in the road haulage and medical sectors providing essential care.

9 June

- Malaysia has reported seven new cases, bringing the total to 8,336. 281 have been discharged, bringing the total number of recoveries to 6,975. There are 1,244 active cases, with six in intensive care and one on ventilator support.
- New Zealand reported no new cases, recoveries, or deaths, which remain at 1,504 (1,154 confirmed and 350 probable), 1,482, and 22 respectively. The country currently has no active cases.

- Singapore has reported 218 new cases, bringing the total to 38,514.
- Ukraine has reported 394 new cases and 13 new deaths, bringing the total numbers to 27,856 and 810, respectively; a total of 12,412 patients have recovered.
- Business Secretary Alok Sharma confirms that all non-essential retailers in England can re-open from Monday 15 June, providing they follow safety guidelines. However, pubs, bars, restaurants, and hairdressers must wait until 4 July "at the earliest" to re-open. Prime Minister Boris Johnson announces that zoos and safari parks will also re-open on 15 June.
- Figures released by the Treasury show that 8.9 million workers are now covered by the Coronavirus Job Retention Scheme, a quarter of the UK workforce, with it having cost £19.6bn to date.
- Thirty medical organisations that represent black, Asian, and minority ethnic doctors and nurses write to Health Secretary Matt Hancock and Equalities Minister Kemi Badenoch expressing their concern at a government review that found black, Asian, and ethnic minority people are twice as likely to die from COVID-19.
- UN Secretary-General António Guterres launched his latest policy brief on the pandemic concerning global food security, emphasizing that the crisis's dire global food security impacts, including an additional 50 million people falling into extreme poverty, could be avoided if countries acted immediately.
- The World Food Programme warned that aid and funding of more than $182 million were urgently required for millions of

people in Nigeria who had been severely impacted by the effects of the coronavirus pandemic, including conflict-hit communities “on life-support” in Nigeria's north-east.

- Hong Kong will allow some students from mainland China to return to resume schooling from June 15 in a selective easing of coronavirus border restrictions. Students will be subjected to temperature screening and submission of health declaration forms in Hong Kong and Shenzhen as they commute to school.
- In Indonesia, the governor of Jakarta, Anies Baswedan, has stated that he is confident that coronavirus is under control. The Indonesian capital can cope with a relaxation of lockdown restrictions that began on June 7.
- Nigeria's Minister of Health Osagie Ehanire up to 60 percent of the "mysterious" deaths reported to authorities in the state of Kano were as a result of the coronavirus.
- President of Tanzania John Magufuli declared Tanzania to be free of the coronavirus.
- In New Delhi, India, authorities have reversed orders limiting the availability of coronavirus testing and reserving hospital beds for city residents after an objection from Prime Minister Narendra Modi.
- The World Health Organization has recommended that Pakistani authorities reimpose "intermittent lockdowns" of targeted areas, stating that the country did not meet the organisation's conditions for lifting restrictions.
- Emirates, the national flag carrier of the United Arab Emirates, has made hundreds of pilots and cabin crew staff redundant, with some reports raising concerns that the company's workforce could potentially be reduced by a third

due to a decline in air travel during the coronavirus pandemic.

- Austria will re-open its border with Italy and more than 20 other European countries next week.
- The Azerbaijani government announced an extension to the country's coronavirus lockdown until July 1. Although borders will remain closed, internal flights will be permitted to resume from June 15.
- French Finance Minister Bruno Le Maire has announced 15 billion euros ($16.9 bn) in rescue money for the aviation industry, including plane manufacturer Airbus and national carrier Air France. Also, in France, the Eiffel Tower will re-open to the public on June 25 after more than three months closed due to the coronavirus lockdown.
- President of Romania Klaus Iohannis stated the need to extend Romania's state of alert to the middle of July. However, this must be approved by the Romanian Parliament to take full effect.
- Turkish President Recep Tayyip Erdoğan has lifted Turkey's stay-at-home orders for people aged over 65 and for children.
- In the United Kingdom, the Office for National Statistics revealed that there had been 64,000 excess deaths in the UK during the coronavirus pandemic. Business Secretary Alok Sharma confirmed that retail outlets will be allowed to open from June 15, with social distancing rules in place.
- In Spain, the Embassy of the United Kingdom in Madrid confirmed that British tourists will be allowed to travel to the country from June 21, although tourists returning to the United Kingdom must undergo a mandatory 14-day

quarantine upon arrival. It was also announced that Spain was in talks with British pharmaceutical company AstraZeneca to make purchases of the company's potential coronavirus vaccine.

- Swedish Health Minister Lena Hallengren has extended the country's ban on visits to nursing homes to the end of August
- In Tajikistan, non-essential businesses, including malls, hotels, and restaurants, re-opened during the first easing of coronavirus lockdown restrictions in the country.
- Non-essential businesses in England, including high-street shops, restaurants, places of worship, and zoos, re-opened with strict social distancing rules in place after being closed for almost two months due to coronavirus lockdown restrictions.
- The regional director for the World Health Organization in the Americas, Carissa Etienne, expressed concerns over surging coronavirus cases across Latin America, including Brazil, Mexico, and Peru.
- In Brazil, a Supreme Federal Court judge has ordered President Jair Bolsonaro to make coronavirus data publicly available after the health ministry removed files from the public domain at the weekend.
- The National Bureau of Economic Research has announced that the United States has officially entered its first recession since 2009.
- Research conducted by Harvard Medical School indicates that COVID-19 could potentially have been spreading in mainland China as early as August 2019. Researchers cited satellite images of hospital movements and search engine

data; Chinese authorities promptly dismissed the claims as "ridiculous."

- Venezuela's Planning Minister Ricardo Menendez reported to state media that flights carrying vital COVID-19 aid from Iran had landed in the country on Monday.

10 June

- Malaysia has reported two new cases, bringing the total to 8,338. 39 patients have recovered, bringing the total number of recoveries to 7,014. There are 1,206 active cases, with five in intensive care.
- New Zealand has reported no new cases, recoveries, or deaths, which remain at 1,504 (1,154 confirmed and 350 probable), 1,482, and 22, respectively. The country currently has no active cases.
- Singapore has reported 451 new cases, bringing the total to 38,965.
- Ukraine has reported 525 new cases and 23 new deaths, bringing the total numbers to 28,381 and 833 respectively; a total of 12,769 patients have recovered.
- Professor Neil Ferguson, the UK government scientist whose advice was crucial in persuading the government to implement the lockdown measures, says that half of the lives lost to COVID-19 could have been saved if the measures had been introduced a week earlier.
- The World Health Organization reported that research was continuing to determine how the COVID-19 virus can be transmitted by people who show no symptoms of the disease.

- Secretary-General António Guterres addressed a virtual gathering of the Global Investors for Sustainable Development Alliance, warning that the "unparalleled economic shock" due to the coronavirus was putting development gains at risk.
- The UN Environment Programme and partners released a new report, Global Trends in Renewable Energy Investment 2020, showing that renewable energy was more cost-effective than ever, as COVID-19 impacted the fossil fuel industry, "providing an opportunity to prioritize clean energy in national economic recovery packages and bring the world closer to meeting the goals of the Paris Agreement."
- Australia's Trade Minister announced that the Australian economy, facing its first recession in thirty years due to the coronavirus, will suffer if Chinese students heeded a warning from their government not to travel to the country because of racist incidents. International education is Australia's fourth-largest foreign exchange earner, worth $26 billion annually. Bill Rawlinson, a senior medical virologist at New South Wales Ministry of Health, said Australia will have largely eradicated the coronavirus by July.
- In the Chinese city of Wuhan, US authorities have announced they will soon resume operations at their consulate based in the city after the US State Department withdrew staff and their families in late January upon the news that the Chinese government would put the city under a lockdown.
- The CEO of the Tokyo 2020 Olympics, Toshiro Muto, has said that the rearranged Olympics will not "be done with grand splendour," but will be simplified. The Games were postponed in March.

- The Africa Centres for Disease Control and Prevention revealed that there had been more than 200,000 confirmed cases of coronavirus in Africa with over 5,000 fatalities.
- Nobel Peace Prize winner Denis Mukwege has resigned as head of a coronavirus task force in an eastern province of the Democratic Republic of the Congo.
- In Malaysia, beauty salons and hairdressers have re-opened after nearly three months of lockdown. The Education Minister also announced that Malaysian schools will begin reopening in stages from June 24. Priority will be given to students taking secondary and equivalent international leaving exams. Students will also have to adhere to social distancing measures and have their temperatures tested when entering schools.
- Sri Lanka will hold parliamentary elections on August 5 after being delayed by three months due to coronavirus restrictions after health authorities gave their approval. Commissioning chairman Mahinda Deshapriya has revealed that a mock election will be held at the weekend to test new health measures that will be implemented at polling booths and counting centres.
- In Austria, Foreign Minister Alexander Schallenberg revealed that from June 16, there will be no checks along the Italian border and no quarantine requirements for more than 20 other European countries.
- Bulgarian Prime Minister Boyko Borisov will extend the country's epidemic emergency to the end of the month in response to a rise in domestically transmitted cases.

- In Denmark, the Japanese company Fujifilm has announced it will spend $928 million to expand the production of COVID-19 treatments in the country.
- Officials at the European Commission have announced their aim to speed up trials for coronavirus vaccines involving genetically modified organisms. Companies including AstraZeneca and Johnson and Johnson have announced they are working on potential COVID-19 vaccines.
- French Finance Minister Bruno Le Maire has said that France could see 800,000 jobs in the aftermath of the pandemic, equivalent to 2.8% of the country's total employment.
- Italian Prime Minister Giuseppe Conte will be questioned by prosecutors on June 12 over his handling of the coronavirus outbreak in northern Italian, one of the country's most badly affected areas. The prosecutors are allegedly investigating why badly hit areas were not closed down faster and have already questioned Lombardy's regional governor and health chief.
- Polish Prime Minister Mateusz Morawiecki has announced that Poland will re-open borders with other European Union countries on June 14 and allow international flights from June 12.
- British Prime Minister Boris Johnson has said that the decision on the timing of the coronavirus lockdown in the UK was based on scientific evidence, in response to Professor Neil Ferguson claiming that Britain's death toll from COVID-19 could have been potentially halved if lockdown had been introduced a week earlier.

- In the United Kingdom, data shows how the British GDP decreased by a record 20.4 percent in April alone as a direct result of restrictions imposed on businesses during the coronavirus pandemic.
- Brazil's most populous state São Paulo has allowed shops to re-open and is preparing to re-open malls, despite Brazil having the third-highest coronavirus death toll in the world. Assembly members in Rio de Janeiro have voted to start an impeachment process against Governor Wilson Witzel on suspected overpricing on purchases of ventilators and other medical supplies to fight the COVID-19 outbreak.
- Flights of Guatemalan migrants from the US will resume twice a week after being suspended due to the coronavirus pandemic.
- Major League Soccer in the United States will resume from July 8 by staging a tournament without spectators, according to MLS Commissioner Don Garber.

11 June

- Brazil has reported a total of 772,416 cases and at least 40,726 deaths.
- Malaysia has reported 31 new cases, bringing the total number to 8,369. 51 cases have been discharged, bringing the total number of recovered to 7,065. There are 1,186 active cases, with five in intensive care.
- New Zealand has reported no new cases, deaths, or recoveries, which remain at a total of 1,504, 22, and 1,482. There are no active cases.

- Singapore has reported 422 new cases, bringing the total to 39,387. In addition, a patient who died from heart disease was subsequently tested positive.
- Ukraine has reported an all-time high of 689 new daily cases as well as 21 new deaths, bringing the total numbers to 29,070 and 854, respectively; a total of 13,141 patients have recovered.
- The United States has reported a total of 2,000,464 cases and 112,908 deaths.
- The UK Health Secretary Matt Hancock describes participation with the Test and Trace programme as a "civic duty".
- Figures from the Office for National Statistics indicate those under the age of 30 have been hardest hit by a fall in income during the COVID-19 outbreak.
- The World Health Organization Africa regional office warned that COVID-19 was accelerating in Africa, with more than 200,000 cases and more than 5,600 deaths.
- Secretary-General António Guterres informed the "High-level Thematic Debate on the Impact of Rapid Technological Change on the Sustainable Development Goals (SDGs) and Targets", taking place in the UN General Assembly, that managing the digital divide better had become "a matter of life and death" owing to people being unable to access essential healthcare information during the pandemic.
- At a virtual roundtable discussion, the Peace Operations chief, Jean-Pierre Lacroix, stressed the importance of prioritizing the UN's Action for Peacekeeping's (A4P) Women, Peace and Security (WPS) commitments during the

pandemic as inequality increased as a result of the pandemic.

- China's Foreign Ministry dismissed a report from the European Union that suggested that Chinese officials were spreading misinformation about the coronavirus.
- According to the Africa Chief of the World Health Organization, the coronavirus pandemic is "accelerating" in the continent, with community transmission reported in more than half of all African countries. Data indicates that it took 18 days for Africa to record 200,000 cases compared to the 98 days it took for the continent to record 100,000 cases.
- Rwanda will receive a further $110 million in economic loans from the International Monetary Fund to assist the country in fighting the coronavirus pandemic. The IMF has now provided Rwanda with over $220 million during the crisis.
- The Malaysian government announced that the country's citizens will not be allowed to make the annual Hajj pilgrimage to Mecca due to concerns over the coronavirus.
- An advisor to the Prime Minister of Pakistan, Imran Khan, announced that Pakistan's GDP is set to contract for the first time in 68 years. Health authorities have also released a statement downplaying a warning to the country from the World Health Organization after the organisation recommended Pakistani officials reimpose a lockdown due to rising cases and death tolls.
- Egyptian authorities announced the reopening of some tourist destinations to international visitors from 1 July in regions of the country with lower coronavirus transmission rates.

- Data from the European Asylum Support Office suggests that applications for asylum in Europe fell 87 percent in April, meaning that the total number of applications is at the lowest level since 2008.
- The French Junior European Affairs Minister Amélie de Montchalin has stated that the 750 billion euro economic recovery package proposed by the European Union must be approved by the end of July, as countries around Europe deal with the financial aftermath of coronavirus lockdowns.
- Airline companies in Norway are now allowed to resume flights at full capacity.
- The British Secretary of State for Health and Social Care Matt Hancock has urged people not to attend Black Lives Matter protests scheduled for the weekend due to the risk of coronavirus transmission. Also, in the UK, Heathrow Airport has started a voluntary redundancy scheme in response to the decline in air travel during the pandemic.
- Turkish-based Pegasus Airlines will resume international flights from 13 June.
- President of Ukraine Volodymyr Zelensky has suspended all official engagements and will restrict his contact with other people after his wife, Olena Zelenska, tested positive for COVID-19.
- The United Nations Conference on Trade and Development announced that international trade is predicted to fall by 27 percent in the second quarter and by 20% annually.
- Passengers on Toronto's public transport system will be required to wear face coverings from 2 July.

- Mayor of Mexico City Claudia Sheinbaum announced an aim of performing 100,000 tests a month at the forefront of the city's plan to ease coronavirus restrictions.
- The United States Department of Labor has revealed that an additional 1.54 million Americans filed for unemployment benefits last week, bringing the total since mid-March to over 44 million. This comes as data from Johns Hopkins University suggests that there are now more than 2 million cases of coronavirus in the US.
- American company Moderna revealed plans to start human trials of its coronavirus vaccines in July.

12 June

- Brazil has reported 909 deaths, bringing the death toll to 41,828. Brazil has reported 25,982 new cases, bringing the total number to 828,810.
- Malaysia has reported 33 new cases, bringing the total number to 8,402. There are 1,115 active cases, with four in intensive care. 103 have been discharged, bringing the number of recovered to 7,168. A new death was recorded, bringing the death toll to 119.
- New Zealand has reported no new cases, deaths, and recoveries, which remain at a total of 1,504, 22, and 1,482. There are no active cases.
- Singapore has reported 463 new cases, bringing the total to 39,850.
- Ukraine has reported 683 new daily cases and 16 new deaths, bringing the total numbers to 29,753 and 870, respectively; a total of 13,567 patients have recovered.

- Figures released by the Office for National Statistics show that the UK economy shrunk by 20.4% in April, the largest monthly contraction on record.
- Further, ONS figures indicate deprived areas have been hit twice as hard by the COVID-19 epidemic when compared to more affluent areas. The impact has also been greater in urban areas compared to rural areas, with London experiencing the highest number of deaths per 100,000.
- The weekly ONS household survey finds that around 33,000 people in England had COVID-19 at any given time between 25 May and 7 June and estimates the rate of new infections to be around 31,600 per week, down from 39,000 the previous week.
- Guy Ryder, Director-General of the International Labour Organization, marking the World Day Against Child Labour, warned that huge gains made towards ending child labour over the previous two decades risked being reversed by the COVID-19 pandemic.
- The UN Children's Fund (UNICEF) warned that children in Yemen, "the world's worst humanitarian disaster," urgently needed basic services, as over eight million Yemenis, nearly half of them children, directly depended on the agency for water, sanitation, and hygiene (WASH) during the ongoing conflict, cholera outbreaks, and pandemic, with the $479 million appeals for Yemen being less than 40 percent funded. UNICEF warned that unless it received $30 million by the end of June, WASH operations for four million people would shut down.

- The World Health Organization warned about the pandemic's impact on women, children, and young people as it continued to escalate.
- Prime Minister of Australia Scott Morrison has urged leaders of the country's states and territories to reopen internal borders to help the Australian economy to recover after coronavirus restrictions were lifted.
- South Korean Health Minister Park Neung-hoo warned that the country's health authorities will extend social distancing rules until newly confirmed cases of coronavirus fall into single figures daily. He also stated that stricter lockdown rules may be re-introduced if newly confirmed cases do not fall to the required level.
- In the Thai capital of Bangkok, the Wat Pho temple, a popular tourist attraction, will not reopen to foreign visitors due to concerns over a potential increase in domestically transmitted cases, although Thai tourists will be permitted to visit the temple.
- Residents of Male, the capital city of the Maldives, will be allowed to travel without permits from 15 June, although gatherings of more than three people remain strictly prohibited.
- Beirut-Rafic Hariri International Airport in Lebanon will reopen to commercial flights from 1 July.
- In Norway, it was announced that travel to Iceland, Finland, and the Swedish island of Gotland will resume from 15 June, although restrictions will remain in place with neighbouring Sweden.

- Spanish Health Minister Salvador Illa announced the state of emergency in the region of Galicia will be lifted on 15 June, making it the first region in the country to do so.
- The World Health Organization stated that coronavirus was affecting the Americas most severely, with the organisation's most senior emergency expert Mike Ryan highlighting how the virus is "highly active" in Latin America.
- Canadian Prime Minister Justin Trudeau announced that it will be mandatory for airline companies to perform temperature checks on all passengers before they arrive in Canada and that passengers with high temperatures will not be permitted to board the flight.
- Governor of Puerto Rico Wanda Vázquez Garced confirmed the reopening of cinemas, gyms, beaches, and churches throughout the territory from 16 June.

13 June

- Malaysia has reported 43 new cases, bringing the total to 8,445. 143 patients have been discharged, bringing the total number of recoveries to 7,311. Health authorities reported a new death, bringing the death toll to 120.
- New Zealand has reported no new cases, deaths, and recoveries, which remain at a total of 1,504, 22, and 1,482. There are no active cases.
- Singapore has reported 347 new cases, bringing the total to 40,197. Another death was later confirmed, bringing the total to 26.
- Ukraine has reported an all-time high of 753 new cases and 10 new deaths, bringing the total numbers to 30,506 and 880, respectively; a total of 13,976 patients have recovered.

- Parts of the Health Protection (Coronavirus, Restrictions) (England) (Amendment No. 4) Regulations 2020 (SI 588) come into effect. In England and Northern Ireland, households with one adult may now become linked with one other household of any size, allowing them to be treated as one for the purpose of permitted gatherings. This also allows the members of one household to stay overnight at the home of the other. The government refers to this as a "support bubble". The rules on gatherings are also relaxed to allow medical appointments and births to be accompanied and to permit some visits to people in hospitals, hospices, and care homes.
- The Welsh Guard performs a unique socially distanced military ceremony at Windsor Castle to mark the Queen's Official Birthday. The ceremony is held in a place of the cancelled Trooping of the Colour and sees the Queen's first public appearance since lockdown began.
- Health officials in the Chinese capital of Beijing closed a street market after the National Health Commission recorded six new domestically transmitted cases, with two of the infected confirmed to have visited the market. Residents in the Fengtai District of Beijing were also placed under lockdown in response to the newly confirmed cases.
- Police in Nepal arrested ten individuals during protests in Kathmandu over the Nepalese government's handling of the coronavirus pandemic.
- In Pakistan, over 1000 coronavirus "hotspots" were sealed off by health authorities in an attempt to control the increasing spread of COVID-19 in the country.

- Researchers in Thailand will test over 100 bats caught in caves for coronavirus to gain a better understanding of the origins of the virus.
- President of Iran Hassan Rouhani announced that the country would reimpose coronavirus lockdown restrictions to prevent another spike of cases in the country if current rules were not followed.
- France will lift all border restrictions with other Schengen countries from 15 June, as well as gradually reopening the country's borders to non-Schengen travellers from 1 July. The news was confirmed by Foreign Minister Jean-Yves Le Drian and Interior Minister Christophe Castaner.
- The Italian Health Minister Roberto Speranza announced that Italy, Germany, France, and the Netherlands have reached an agreement with British pharmaceutical company AstraZeneca to supply 400 million doses of the company's coronavirus vaccines at the cost of over $800 million, with the aim of the first doses being prescribed by the end of 2020. AstraZeneca further revealed that it had entered discussions with health authorities in Brazil, China, Japan, and Russia regarding the supply of the company's coronavirus vaccine.
- British-based airline EasyJet announced that some domestic flights in the UK would resume from 15 June.
- In Gaborone, the capital city of Botswana, the government has re-introduced a strict coronavirus lockdown after twelve new cases of the virus were confirmed in the city's hospitals.
- Chile's Minister of Health, Jaime Mañalich, was replaced due to controversies surrounding the country's reporting of coronavirus cases.

- Mayor of Mexico City Claudia Sheinbaum has revealed her plans to ease coronavirus lockdown restrictions in the city. Public transport and cars will be allowed to return to the roads from next week, and markets, shopping centres, restaurants, and places of worship will be permitted to reopen a week later at reduced capacities. Some of Mexico's administrative regions that have falling numbers of cases of coronavirus, as well as an acceptable number of spare hospital beds, will permit the gradual reopening of hotels and other leisure facilities from 22 June.
- The economic adviser to US President Donald Trump, Larry Kudlow, stated that Trump's administration is not concerned about a potential second wave of coronavirus in the country.

14 June

- China has reported 57 new cases, including 36 in Beijing.
- Malaysia has reported eight new cases (two imported and six local transmissions), bringing the total to 8,453. 35 patients have recovered, bringing the total number of recoveries to 7,346. 1 new death was recorded, bringing the death toll to 121.
- New Zealand has reported no new cases, deaths, and recoveries, which remain at a total of 1,504, 22, and 1,482. There are no active cases.
- Singapore has reported 407 new cases, bringing the total to 40,604.
- Ukraine has reported 648 new cases and 9 new deaths, bringing the total numbers to 31,154 and 889, respectively; a total of 14,082 patients have recovered.

- In response to an outbreak resulting in dozens of news cases in Beijing, authorities in Beijing have stepped testing, contact tracing, ordered companies to impose a 14-day quarantine for employees who have visited the Xinfadi market, and locked down neighbourhoods.
- A regular China Southern Airlines flight between Dhaka and Guangzhou will be suspended for four weeks from 22 June after passengers from the flight on 11 June tested positive for COVID-19.
- In the Indian capital of New Delhi, 500 railway coaches will serve as field hospitals, and authorities will conduct house-to-house health surveys to attempt to control the increasing spread of the coronavirus in the city.
- All airports in Egypt will reopen from 1 July, according to the country's Aviation Minister.
- In Oman, a committee has been formed by the Sultan to address the economic consequences of the coronavirus pandemic in the country.
- In the Saudi Arabian capital of Riyadh, the embassies of Yemen and the Philippines will both close temporarily for disinfecting after a number of staff in both buildings tested positive for coronavirus.
- Austrian Economy Minister Margarete Schramböck revealed that the country plans to introduce further investment subsidies and tax breaks to help struggling businesses deal with the effects of the coronavirus pandemic.
- President of France Emmanuel Macron announced that all of mainland France, including the capital Paris, will enter a lower state of alert on 15 June, meaning that restaurants and cafés can operate in normal circumstances.

- Spain will reopen its borders to countries in the Schengen Area from 21 June without the need for tourists to undergo a mandatory quarantine upon arrival. The border with Portugal will reopen later on 1 July.
- British Chancellor of the Exchequer Rishi Sunak announced that the government will review the 2-metre social distancing rule currently in place in the UK, over reports that suggest that millions of jobs could be saved if the distance was reduced, similar to other countries around the world. This comes as the European Director of the World Health Organization, Hans Kluge, warned that coronavirus lockdown measures in England should not be lifted further until the government's contact tracing scheme is operating more successfully.
- Chile's Finance Minister has revealed an economic stimulus package worth $12 billion to assist the country in mitigating the effects on the economy of the coronavirus pandemic.
- President of El Salvador Nayib Bukele announced that the country's economy could potentially reopen in stages from 16 June, although the country's main airport will not reopen until 6 August.
- In the US, players and staff in the National Basketball Association will be tested for COVID-19 every two days before the season resumes in Orlando from 23 June.
- Sudan's airports will not reopen for another two weeks until 28 June at the earliest.

15 June

- Malaysia has reported 41 new cases, bringing the total to 8,494. 54 have been discharged, bringing the total number of recovered patients to 7,400. There are currently 973 active cases. The death toll remains at 121.
- New Zealand has reported no new cases, deaths, and recoveries, which remain at a total of 1,504, 22, and 1,482. There are currently no active cases.
- Singapore has reported 214 new cases, bringing the total to 40,818.
- Ukraine has reported 656 new cases and 12 new deaths, bringing the total numbers to 31,810 and 901, respectively; a total of 14,253 patients have recovered.
- The remainder of the Health Protection (Coronavirus, Restrictions) (England) (Amendment No. 4) Regulations 2020 (SI 588) comes into effect, allowing the general reopening of English retail shops and public-facing businesses apart from those that are on a list of specific exclusions such as restaurants, bars, pubs, nightclubs, most cinemas, theatres, museums, hairdressers, indoor sports and leisure facilities. Outdoor animal-related attractions such as farms, zoos and safari parks may open. Places of worship may again be used for private prayer (but not for communal worship). English libraries still have to remain closed.
- The Isle of Man lifts restrictions on social distancing except in health and care environments.
- Wearing a face covering becomes mandatory on public transport.

- India reimposed lockdowns in Chennai and other areas in the state of Tamil Nadu due to a rise in coronavirus cases.
- Malaysian Senior Minister Ismail Sabri Yaakob announced that all 5,230 non-Muslim places of worship would be allowed to reopen but would have to implement social distancing guidelines, including taking one-third of their usual capacity and requiring attendees to download the MySejahtera application.
- The World Health Organization Director-General, Tedros Adhanom Ghebreyesus, emphasized the risk of the southern hemisphere influenza season, as "Co-circulation of COVID-19 and influenza can worsen the impact on health systems that are already overwhelmed".
- A further ten neighbourhoods in the Haidian District of the Chinese capital, Beijing, were placed into lockdown after a sudden rise in infections linked to a wholesale market were reported to authorities.
- Hong Kong Disneyland announced that the attraction will reopen to visitors on 18 June.
- Japan's Ministry of Foreign Affairs said the Japanese government had not made a decision to ease the country's coronavirus entry ban.
- President of the Philippines Rodrigo Duterte confirmed that some coronavirus lockdown restrictions would remain in place in Manila for a further two weeks, whilst also reimposing a full lockdown in Cebu City due to a rise in cases.
- In Singapore, the government announced that most businesses will be allowed to reopen from 19 June.

- The World Health Organization and UNICEF released a joint report warning that over 50,000 children in the Middle East and North Africa could die from coronavirus.
- In the Industrial Area of the Qatari capital of Doha, the necessity for entry and exit permits has been removed by authorities. Qatar also entered the first phase of easing coronavirus lockdown restrictions, whereby some non-essential shops and places of worship may be allowed to reopen.
- Authorities in the United Arab Emirates announced that residents will be permitted to travel to specific locations from 23 June, although the capital Abu Dhabi extended a ban restricting movements in and out of the city for an additional week. Authorities also announced that residents will be allowed to travel to countries deemed by the government to be low-risk for coronavirus transmission from 23 June.
- Prime Minister of Finland Sanna Marin announced that the emergency powers adopted by the Finnish Parliament would be withdrawn due to falling coronavirus cases in the country. The country's state of emergency ended at midnight.
- In Greece, major international airports have reopened to foreign tourists, although passengers arriving from countries deemed high-risk by the European Union will have to undergo a mandatory 14-day quarantine. Bans on travellers from the UK and Turkey were extended to 30 June.
- North Macedonia's general election has been rescheduled to 15 July after being delayed due to coronavirus restrictions in the country.

- Chile's government extended the country's "state of catastrophe" measures by 90 days in response to rapidly increasing numbers of coronavirus cases.
- Governor of New York Andrew Cuomo revealed that parts of New York City in a lower state of emergency will permit gatherings of up to 25 people.
- The US Food and Drug Administration reversed its decision to allow emergency authorisation for the malaria drug hydroxychloroquine after its effectiveness in treating COVID-19 was questioned by scientists.
- Organisers of the 2021 Academy Awards announced that the date of the ceremony had been pushed back to 25 April from the original scheduled date of 28 February as a result of coronavirus concerns.

16 June

- China has reported 40 new cases, including 27 in Beijing. The capital has reported a total of 106 cases.
- Malaysia has reported 11 new cases (10 local transmissions and one imported), bringing the total to 8,505. There have been 333 recoveries, bringing the total number of recovered patients to 7,733. The death toll remains at 121.
- New Zealand has reported two new active cases (both imported), bringing the total number of combined cases to 1,506 (1,156 confirmed and 350 probable). The total number of recovered and deaths remain at 1,482 and 22 respectively. These two new cases break the 24 consecutive days of no new cases in the country.
- Singapore has reported 151 new cases, bringing the total to 40,969.

- Ukraine has reported 666 new cases and 11 new deaths, bringing the total numbers to 32,476 and 912, respectively; a total of 14,528 patients have recovered.
- The low-dose steroid treatment dexamethasone, which has been part of clinical trials for existing drugs that could be used to treat patients with COVID-19, is heralded as a major breakthrough after it was found to cut the number of deaths. Experts estimate up to 5,000 lives may have been saved in the UK had the treatment been used from the outset. Prime Minister Boris Johnson describes the news as a genuine case to celebrate "a remarkable British scientific achievement". Dexamethasone will be made available through the NHS, which has a stockpile of 200,000 doses.
- Office for National Statistics figures suggests more than 600,000 people have lost their jobs between March and May because of the impact of the COVID-19 outbreak.
- A report published by National Foundation for Educational Research (NFER) suggests that 90% of teachers say their pupils are doing less work than would be the usual case for the time of year, while headteachers say a third of pupils are not engaging with the work set for them by their teachers.
- Pakistan's health authorities will implement strict coronavirus lockdowns in certain neighbourhoods of twenty cities found to be at an increased risk of an accelerated spread of the virus.
- The UNHCR warned of the worsening refugee crisis in Syria, as "another 200,000 refugees just in this period of three months who because of the impact needed emergency assistance".

- The UN's office for Latin America and the Caribbean (ECLAC), together with the Food and Agriculture Organization, proposed in a new study 10 measures to avoid increased hunger in the region, including through an "anti-hunger grant", as they warned those living in extreme poverty in the region could surpass 83 million by the end of 2020 due to the impacts of the pandemic.
- In the Chinese capital of Beijing, schools have been forced to close in response to a new outbreak of coronavirus at a wholesale market in the city, and more neighbourhoods surrounding the Haidian District have been placed under lockdown in response to the outbreak, with half of Beijing's districts reporting new cases. In the city of Shanghai, travellers from regions in China deemed to be at a medium or high risk of coronavirus will have to undergo a mandatory 14-day quarantine upon arrival.
- Hong Kong's Department of Health announced that groups of up to fifty people will be allowed from 19 June.
- Schools in regions of Indonesia deemed to be at a lower risk of coronavirus will begin a phased reopening in July.
- Air New Zealand announced that it would be resuming flights between Auckland and Shanghai from 22 June. That same day, the New Zealand Government suspended compassionate exemptions for travelers after two women who had visited the country in June to attend a funeral tested positive for COVID-19.
- In Singapore, scientists at Duke-NUS Medical School will begin clinical trials of a potential coronavirus vaccine in August after successful trials on animals.

- The charity Amnesty International expressed its concerns over potential privacy breaches involving the coronavirus contact tracing apps used by Kuwait and Bahrain.
- Authorities in Denmark have encouraged Black Lives Matter protestors in Copenhagen to get tested for COVID-19 after a protestor tested positive for the virus.
- Members of Hungary's National Assembly voted in favour of revoking emergency powers granted to Prime Minister Viktor Orbán during the coronavirus pandemic.
- Turkish Health Minister Fahrettin Koca announced that it will be mandatory to wear face coverings in 42 provinces of the country.
- The wife of the President of Ukraine, Olena Zelenska, has been admitted to the hospital in a stable condition after testing positive for COVID-19.
- In the United Kingdom, researchers at the University of Oxford published the results of studies involving the drug dexamethasone, suggesting that the drug can cause significant reductions of up to a third in coronavirus mortality rates amongst patients who require ventilator treatment, making it the first successful treatment to be found for coronavirus in the world. On the same day, the Medicines and Healthcare products Regulatory Agency instructed human trials involving the malaria drug hydroxychloroquine to cease immediately after growing concerns amongst the international community over the effectiveness of the drug in treating COVID-19.
- In the UK, it was reported that more than 600,000 citizens have lost their jobs during the country's coronavirus lockdown, with the number of people claiming

unemployment benefits rising by over 23 per cent to 2.8 million.

- Carissa Etienne, the regional director for the World Health Organization in the Americas, warned in a press conference that the COVID-19 pandemic is still accelerating in both continents.
- The USA's border closures with Canada and Mexico were extended to 21 July.
- Airlines in the US will reportedly ban passengers who refuse to wear a face-covering on their flight.
- Organisers of the 2020 US Open tennis tournament confirmed that the event would go ahead as scheduled on 31 August, although all matches will be played without spectators.
- The 2020 Western Idaho Fair, the largest event in the state, was cancelled for the first time since 1935 due to the pandemic, but in return to its roots and for the sake of manageable public health logistics plans to scale drastically down solely to 4-H and Future Farmers of America youth exhibits, competitions and sales.

17 June

- Malaysia has reported ten new cases (all local transmissions), bringing the total to 8,515. There are 642 active aces with four in intensive care. 140 patients have been discharged, bringing the total number of recoveries to 7,873. The death toll remains at 121.
- New Zealand has two active cases (both imported), bringing the total number of combined cases to 1,506 (1,156 confirmed and 350 probable). The total number of recovered

and deaths remain at 1,482 and 22 respectively. That same day, the Ministry of Health announced that it had identified 320 people who had been in contact with the two new cases.

- Singapore has reported 247 new cases, bringing the total to 41,216.
- Ukraine sets a new record for both daily cases and deaths at 758 and 31, respectively. The totals are now 33,234 cases and 943 lethal outcomes. Additionally, 14,943 patients have recovered overall.
- Canada tops 100.000 cases
- Speaking to the Science and Technology Committee, Lord Bethell, the Minister for Innovation at the Department of Health and Social Care, says the contact tracing app is "not a priority" and may not be ready until the winter.
- Health Secretary Matt Hancock is pictured slapping a colleague on the back as they arrived at the House of Commons for Prime Minister's Questions, apparently forgetting social distancing measures.
- The World Health Organization welcomed early results on the use of dexamethasone in sickest COVID-19 patients while warning it's 'no cure-all'.
- New Zealand Prime Minister Jacinda Ardern announced that the New Zealand Defence Force's Assistant Chief of Defence Air commodore Darryn Webb will oversee the country's border and quarantine isolation facilities after two women, who had been granted compassionate exemptions to attend a funeral, tested positive for COVID-19 the previous day.
- A government-led study in Tunisia found that the country's economy could potentially shrink by as much as 6.7 per cent

as a direct result of coronavirus restrictions, with 275,000 people expected to lose their jobs.

- The Russian government announced that foreign athletes would be able to enter the country to participate in domestic sports competitions.
- Prime Minister of the United Kingdom Boris Johnson warned there could potentially never be a vaccine for COVID-19.
- Developers behind Germany's coronavirus contact tracing app announced that it has been downloaded 6.5 million times since its launch on 16 June. On the same day, German company CureVac announced that it was ready to begin clinical trials of a potential coronavirus vaccine, becoming the second company in the country to do so. Chancellor of Germany Angela Merkel also extended the country's ban on large events to October.
- Portugal's Assembly of the Republic voted to increase the government's budget by 4.3 billion euros to aid the country's recovery from the coronavirus pandemic.
- Prime Minister of Spain Pedro Sánchez announced that the country's 27,000 coronavirus victims would be honoured in a state ceremony on 16 July.
- Swedish Minister for Foreign Affairs Ann Linde announced that Sweden will allow residents to travel for non-essential reasons to ten countries in the European Union from 30 June, including France, Italy, and Spain.
- The Premier League in England resumed without spectators after previously being suspended due to coronavirus concerns, with police urging fans not to gather outside stadiums.

- Mayor of London Sadiq Khan announced he would be taking a 10 per cent pay cut in response to London's struggling financial situation as a result of the pandemic.
- Researchers at Israel's Technion Institute of Technology in Haifa revealed that they had invented a reusable face mask capable of killing the coronavirus with heat by utilising the power from a mobile phone charger, the first such face mask produced worldwide.
- Mining companies in the Democratic Republic of the Congo will receive financial support from the government to ease the economic consequences of the coronavirus pandemic.
- In Chile's capital of Santiago, the government imposed tighter lockdown restrictions meaning that people are only permitted to leave their homes twice a week with heavy fines if caught breaking the rules, in response to the country recording over 200,000 cases of coronavirus.
- President of Honduras Juan Orlando Hernández announced that he had tested positive for COVID-19 and would subsequently work from home.
- In the United States, the Navajo Nation reimposed a strict lockdown for its citizens over the weekend in response to increasing cases of coronavirus in bordering Arizona.

18 June

- Malaysia has reported 14 new cases, bringing the total to 8,529. There are 408 active cases, with four in intensive care. 127 have recovered, bringing the total number of recoveries to 8,000. The death toll remains at 119.
- New Zealand has reported one new case, bringing the number of active cases to three and the total number to

1,507 (1,157 confirmed and 350 probable). The new case is a man in his sixties who traveled from Pakistan to Doha to Melbourne on 11 June before flying from Melbourne to Auckland on 13 June. A total of 327,460 people have been tested in New Zealand, with 6,273 tested on 18 June.

- Singapore has reported 257 new cases, bringing the total to 41,473.
- Ukraine sets a new record for daily cases at 829 and reports 23 new deaths. The totals are now 34,063 cases and 966 lethal outcomes. Additionally, 15,447 patients have recovered overall.
- The Bank of England announces plans to inject an extra £100bn into the UK economy to help fight the downturn precipitated by the pandemic.
- The UK delays the launch of the contact tracing app and changes its original format in favour of a model based on technology designed by Apple and Google. Compatibility issues were found between the app's and Apple's software, but unlike Apple's model, the UK app is able to better measure distance, so the plan is to combine aspects of both into a single app. The Apple-Google model is also less centralised but more secure.
- The weekly ONS household survey estimates that around 33,000 people in England had COVID-19 at any given time between 31 May and 13 June, unchanged from the previous week. Antibodies were found in 5.4% of 1,757 people who gave blood samples since 26 April.
- Health Secretary Matt Hancock announces that pharmaceutical company AstraZeneca and Oxford University have reached a deal to begin the manufacture of a potential

vaccine, even though it has yet to receive clinical approval. The plan is to stockpile the vaccine ready for its approval. Those over the age of 50 and with certain underlying health conditions will then be prioritised for the vaccine once launched.

- Office for National Statistics data for the two weeks up to 10 June indicates that of the 14,000 names passed to NHS Test and Trace for follow up, 10,200 had been contacted.
- Australian national carrier Qantas announced that most international flights scheduled before October had been cancelled after the Australian government suggested that the country's borders may be closed until 2021.
- Prime Minister of Japan Shinzo Abe announced that travellers from Australia, New Zealand, Thailand, and Vietnam will be allowed to enter the country in the coming weeks.
- New Zealand Director-general of Health Ashley Bloomfield announced that all travelers on trans-Tasman flights will be required to wear face masks in response to three new imported cases resulting from overseas travel.
- Thailand's aviation authorities stated that international travel to the country may be allowed to resume from July if cases continue to fall.
- The Jordanian government revealed the results of a study suggesting that the country's unemployment rate could rise to 19 per cent and that the economy could shrink by as much as 3.5 per cent in 2020 due to the pandemic. A report from the United Nations also found that many citizens were struggling to meet basic needs.

- The government of Kuwait announced that from 21 June, curfew hours will be eased and that residents with critical health conditions will be allowed to travel freely around the country. The government also said that the current Phase 1 of reopening would remain in place for an additional week.
- The CEO of Qatar Airways, Akbar Al Baker, revealed that the company would not make purchases of any new aircraft until 2022 as a result of the financial consequences of the coronavirus pandemic.
- Czech Health Minister Adam Vojtěch announced that restrictions imposed due to coronavirus will be eased in the coming weeks to allow larger groups of people to gather and leisure attractions to reopen, as well as remove the necessity to wear face masks.
- Denmark will allow citizens from Schengen countries to travel to the country from 27 June, although Portugal and Sweden won't be included due to having higher rates of infection.
- The Federal Statistical Office of Germany found that the German travel industry declined by 23 per cent in the first quarter of 2020, making it the largest decline since the 2008 Financial Crisis.
- In Kazakhstan, non-essential shops, markets, and public parks will be closed from 21 June as a result of increasing cases of coronavirus. This comes as former President of Kazakhstan Nursultan Nazarbayev tested positive for COVID-19.
- The Slovenian government announced that all travellers arriving in the country from Serbia, Kosovo, and Bosnia

would have to undergo a mandatory 14-day quarantine due to an increase in transmissions in the country.

- The Spanish tourism industry will receive a 4.25 billion euro stimulus package to aid recovery from the pandemic.
- Swedish Finance Minister Magdalena Andersson revealed that the country's economy is predicted to decrease by six per cent in 2020 due to the coronavirus pandemic.
- The British government announced that the country would switch to using a contact tracing app developed by Google and Apple after trials of the country's own app on the Isle of Wight highlighted significant problems with identifying Apple phones.
- Swiss authorities announced that gatherings of up to 1000 people will be allowed from 22 June.
- In the United Kingdom, the coronavirus alert level was lowered from Level 4 to Level 3, meaning that transmission of the virus is no longer rising.
- As the country entered the final day of its state of alert introduced in March to control the spread of coronavirus.
- Swiss pharmaceutical company Novartis announced it would stop trials of the malaria drug hydroxychloroquine for potential COVID-19 treatment due to a lack of volunteers for clinical trials and data from the World Health Organization raising questions over the effectiveness of the drug.
- Turkish health authorities have imposed a nationwide curfew between 9 am and 3 pm every day to reduce the spread of coronavirus whilst high school entry exams are being conducted.
- Chinese Communist Party general secretary Xi Jinping announced that some countries in Africa will not have to

repay zero-interest-rate loans paid by China before the end of the year to aid the continent's recovery from the coronavirus.

- President of the United States Donald Trump stated that the US would not reimpose lockdown restrictions despite a number of states reporting surges in coronavirus cases, highlighting the huge economic consequences such a measure would have.
- The United States Department of Labor revealed that a further 1.5 million Americans filed for unemployment in the last week, bringing the country's total number of people who have lost their jobs during the pandemic to over 45 million.
- Health authorities in the US state of California introduced a new law requiring all residents to wear face coverings outside of their homes.
- Mayor of New York Bill de Blasio announced that the city will move into the second phase of reopening on 22 June after months of coronavirus lockdown restrictions. Non-essential businesses, including hairdressers and offices, will be allowed to reopen as part of the easing of restrictions.

19 June

- Brazil reaches 1 million cases worldwide.
- Malaysia has reported six new cases, bringing the total number to 8,535. There are 344 active cases, with four in intensive care. 70 have recovered, bringing the total number of recovered to 8,070. The death toll remains at 121. That same day, the Director-General Noor Hisham Abdullah confirmed the discovery of a new cluster in Kidurong, Sarawak.

- New Zealand has reported no new cases, with the total number of active cases remaining at three. A total of 327,460 people have been tested in New Zealand. The total number of cases remains 1,507 (1,157 confirmed and 350 probable).
- Singapore has reported 142 new cases, bringing the total to 41,615.
- Ukraine sets a new record for daily cases at 921 and reports 19 new deaths. The totals are now 34,984 cases and 985 lethal outcomes. Additionally, 16,033 patients have recovered overall.
- The UK's COVID-19 Alert Level is lowered from Level 4 (severe risk, high transmission) to Level 3 (substantial risk, general circulation), following the agreement of all four Chief Medical Officers. Health Secretary Matt Hancock describes the change as "a big moment for the country".
- Figures from the Treasury show that UK debt stands at £1.95trn and is larger than the economy for the first time in 50 years following a record amount of borrowing in May. The amount borrowed in May was £55.2bn, nine times higher than borrowing for May 2019, and the highest monthly amount since records began.
- The World Health Organization warned that the world was entering "a new and dangerous phase" of the COVID-19 pandemic, as infection rates continued to climb and over 150,000 new cases of the disease were reported the previous day, the highest single daily total to date.
- Secretary-General António Guterres issued a new policy brief, the World of Work and COVID-19, concerning jobs, livelihoods, and the well-being of workers, families, and

businesses globally, as they continued to be affected by the COVID-19 pandemic; with micro, small and medium enterprises, in particular, suffering dire economic consequences.

- Authorities in Beijing stated that the coronavirus outbreak in the city was under control after a sudden increase in cases linked to a wholesale market was reported over a week ago. Authorities also revealed that a potential coronavirus vaccine being developed by Chinese company Clover Biopharmaceuticals had reached clinical trials on human volunteers.
- Shinzo Abe announced that all domestic travel restrictions in Japan would be lifted with immediate effect, with residents actively encouraged to engage in leisure activities that will aid the country's economic recovery from the pandemic.
- In Singapore, non-essential businesses, including gyms and restaurants, reopened, with gatherings of up to five people also permitted.
- Mosques in the Saudi Arabian city of Mecca were announced to be reopening from 21 June after being closed three months ago due to the pandemic.
- Germany's coronavirus contact tracing app has been downloaded almost 10 million times, according to government data.
- Ireland's Taoiseach Leo Varadkar revealed that, from 29 June, churches, hairdressers and gyms will be allowed to reopen, with gatherings of up to 200 people outdoors and 50 people indoors also permitted. On the same date, all sporting activities will resume, and the government is expected to provide 70 million euros in economic support to

businesses affected by the pandemic. Varadkar also announced that the country's mandatory 14-day quarantine for anybody arriving in the country would remain in place until at least 9 July.

- Deputy Prime Minister of Poland Jadwiga Emilewicz announced that airline companies will be allowed to operate flights at full capacity from 1 July.
- In Zimbabwe, Health Minister Obadiah Moyo was arrested for alleged corruption regarding the country's supply of protective equipment needed to combat the coronavirus outbreak. He will appear in court on 20 June.
- Costa Rica's Health Minister Daniel Salas announced that the country's reopening programme would be temporarily paused in response to a rise in cases of coronavirus.
- Health Minister of Guatemala Hugo Monroy and three of his deputies were replaced by President of Guatemala Alejandro Giammattei.
- Mayor of the District of Columbia Muriel Bowser announced that Washington D.C. will enter the second phase of its reopening plan next week, which will allow non-essential shops and restaurants to operate indoors with strict social distancing guidelines.

20 June

- Malaysia has reported 21 new cases, bringing the total to 8,556. There are 289 active cases, with three cases in intensive care. 76 have recovered, bringing the total number of recoveries to 8,146. The death toll remains at 121.
- New Zealand has reported two new asymptomatic cases, bringing the number of active cases to five. This brings the

total number of cases to 1,509 (1,159 confirmed and 350 probable).

- Singapore has reported 218 new cases, bringing the total to 41,833.
- Ukraine has reported 841 new cases and 9 new deaths, bringing the total numbers to 35,825 and 994, respectively; a total of 16,406 patients have recovered.
- Culture Secretary Oliver Dowden and Chancellor Rishi Sunak confirm that the review into the 2m social distancing rule in England will conclude within the coming days.
- Spain's foreign affairs minister Arancha González Laya announces that UK tourists will be able to visit Spain without the need for quarantine from the following day.
- Guernsey lifts the majority of its lockdown restrictions, meaning social distancing measures are no longer required, and pubs, restaurants, and other businesses can operate at normal capacity. But border controls remain in place.
- Northern Ireland records 1 death in the most recent 24 hour period, but no new cases of COVID-19 for the first time since March.
- In Australia, Premier of Victoria, Daniel Andrews, announced that the state would reimpose some restrictions after sustained rises in coronavirus cases. Andrews revealed that as part of the tightened restrictions, outdoor gatherings will be limited to ten people and that areas that are deemed to be hotspots for the virus could have stricter restrictions imposed.
- The United States Department of State revealed that a number of employees of the American Embassy in Afghanistan's capital city of Kabul had tested positive for

coronavirus and that the embassy was taking measures to prevent further transmission of the virus.

- International flights to and from Pakistan resumed after being suspended for over three months due to coronavirus.
- Prime Minister of the State of Palestine Mohammad Shtayyeh announced that the cities of Hebron and Nablus would be closed to prevent the further spread of coronavirus.
- Authorities in Saudi Arabia confirmed that the country's curfew would be lifted on 21 June and that all economic activity would be allowed to continue.
- In France, it was announced that football stadiums will be allowed to reopen to a maximum of 5,000 spectators from 11 July.
- Prime Minister of Kyrgyzstan Kubatbek Boronov announced that all public transport would cease in the capital city of Bishkek due to a rise in coronavirus cases in the city.
- President of Montenegro Milo Đukanović announced that the country's general election had been scheduled for 30 August due to Montenegro having relatively few cases of the virus.
- Spanish Foreign Minister Arancha González Laya announced that British tourists would be permitted to enter the country from 21 June without having to undergo a mandatory 14-day quarantine upon arrival, although any travellers arriving in the UK must still enter self-isolation. The decision was said to have been d "out of respect" for the 400,000 British citizens with homes in Spain. Prime Minister of Spain Pedro Sánchez urged the population to be cautious.
- The United Nations Special Representative in Haiti Helen La Lime warned that the coronavirus pandemic is worsening Haiti's humanitarian situation, stating that the country was in

desperate need of financial aid from the international community to stimulate the economy.

- Mayor of Mexico City Claudia Sheinbaum announced that authorities had postponed a planned reopening of the city's economy due to rising numbers of cases and a high rate of hospital bed occupancy.

21 June

- Malaysia has reported 16 new cases, bringing the total number to 8,572. There are 295 active cases, with three in intensive care. The death toll remains at 121. Ten patients have recovered, bringing the total number of recoveries to 8,156.
- New Zealand has reported two new cases, bringing the number of active cases to seven. There are a total of 1,511 (1,161 confirmed and 350 probable) cases. The number of recovered remains at 1,482, and the death toll remains at 22.
- Singapore has reported 262 new cases, bringing the total to 42,095.
- Ukraine has reported 735 new cases and 8 new deaths, bringing the total numbers to 36,560 and 1,002, respectively; a total of 16,509 patients have recovered.
- The US state of Florida has reported 3,494 new cases, bringing the total in the state to 97. The state's death toll has reached 3,161.
- No new COVID-19 deaths are recorded for Scotland and Northern Ireland.

- Health authorities in the Australian state of Victoria announced that the state of emergency would be extended to 19 July due to a rise in coronavirus infections.
- Chinese health officials announced that frozen meat imports from American company Tyson Foods would be suspended indefinitely after positive cases of COVID-19 were reported at the company's factory in the US. A PepsiCo factory in Beijing was also ordered to close after employees tested positive. This comes as authorities in Beijing revealed that the city now had the capacity to test 1 million people a day for coronavirus.
- Researchers at the Peking Union Medical College announced that they have started the second phase of human trials for a potential coronavirus vaccine.
- Authorities in Saudi Arabia lifted the country's coronavirus lockdown and allowed businesses, including hairdressers and cinemas, to reopen. The Ministry of Tourism of Saudi Arabia also announced plans to launch a $4 billion tourism development fund to stimulate the country's economy.
- In the United Arab Emirates, international visitors will be permitted to travel to Dubai from 7 July, with all travellers required to provide evidence of a negative test for COVID-19 or be tested at the airport.
- The final of the Adria Tour tennis tournament was cancelled after Bulgarian player Grigor Dimitrov tested positive for COVID-19.
- Police in the Dutch city of The Hague reportedly arrested multiple individuals who refused to leave protests over the government's social distancing rules.

- Spain's borders were reopened to international tourists from the United Kingdom and all Schengen countries, with the exception of Portugal. The country's state of emergency imposed in March as a result of coronavirus was lifted.
- In the United Kingdom, Chancellor of the Exchequer Rishi Sunak revealed plans to cut Value-added tax (VAT) to reduce the economic impact of the coronavirus pandemic.
- President of the United States Donald Trump told supporters at a rally in Tulsa, Oklahoma, that he had asked health authorities to slow down the rate of testing for COVID-19. A spokesperson from the White House later stated that Trump had been "joking".
- In Morocco, a new field hospital was set up to treat more infected people amid a surge in cases in the country.

22 June

- Malaysia has reported 15 new cases, bringing the total number of cases to 8,587. There are 289 active cases, with two in intensive care. 21 cases have been discharged, bringing the total number of recovered to 8,177. The death toll remains at 121.
- New Zealand has reported two new cases, bringing the total number of active cases to nine. There are a total of 1,513 cases (1,163 confirmed cases and 350 probable cases). The number of recovered and death toll remains at 1,482 and 22 respectively.
- Singapore has reported 218 new cases, bringing the total to 42,313.

- Ukraine has reported 681 new cases and 10 new deaths, bringing the total numbers to 37,241 and 1,012, respectively; a total of 16,642 patients have recovered.
- A new coronavirus saliva test is trialled in the UK.
- The UK records its lowest number of new coronavirus cases since the beginning of lockdown, with 958 people have tested positive for the virus, the first time the figure has dropped below 1,000; the number of deaths recorded for the previous day stands at 15, the lowest figure since 15 March.
- The energy regulator Ofgem gives energy companies permission to follow up unpaid bills, but warns them not to be aggressive in their pursuit of unpaid debts.
- The World Health Organization reported the largest single-day increase in coronavirus cases over 21 June, registering more than 183,000 new infections in 24 hours, with approximately 8.8 million cases in total worldwide, with more than 465,000 deaths.
- UNAIDS warned that stocks of medication for HIV patients could be exhausted within the next two months due to higher costs as a result of lockdowns and COVID-19 border closures.
- New Zealand Prime Minister Jacinda Ardern has announced that the New Zealand Government would require people to test negative for COVID-19 before leaving quarantine. The government also extended the ban on cruise ships beyond 30 June. While cargo ships and fishing vessels will be allowed to dock, and ship crew arriving in New Zealand would need to spend 14 days in quarantine if they had not been on the vessel for 28 days prior to docking.

- Mayor of Seoul Park Won-soon announced that city authorities would impose stricter measures if the number of new daily infections did not fall below thirty in the coming days. This comes as South Korean officials stated that the country was experiencing a second wave of infections.
- Authorities in Saudi Arabia announced that a "very limited" Hajj would take place in July, with the pilgrimage to Mecca being exclusively for Saudi residents due to fears of coronavirus transmission if a large number of pilgrims were to attend.
- In the United Arab Emirates, Abu Dhabi announced that residents can now move freely between cities in the emirate from 23 June and extended restrictions for non-residents entering the city.
- Bulgarian Health Minister Kiril Ananiev announced that it would again be mandatory to wear face masks in indoor public spaces after a large increase in coronavirus cases in the country.
- Disneyland Paris announced it would be partially reopening from 15 July with reduced visitor numbers and the requirement to wear face masks.
- French Finance Minister Bruno Le Maire revealed that French and German authorities were calling for the European Recovery Fund to pay out the proposed 500 billion euros of financial aid until 2022 rather than until 2024, which was suggested by other member states.
- Prime Minister of Portugal António Costa announced that some coronavirus restrictions would be reimposed in the capital Lisbon from 23 June, with new restrictions limiting

social gatherings to ten people and requirements for shops and restaurants to close before 8pm.

- Health officials in the United Kingdom announced that a saliva test for coronavirus would be trialled in Southampton with the aim of identifying outbreaks faster.
- The organisers of the 2021 Golden Globe Awards announced that the date of the ceremony had been pushed back to 28 February due to the coronavirus pandemic.
- In New York City, restaurants reopened outdoor seating areas, and retail outlets were also permitted to reopen.

23 June

- Malaysia has reported three new cases, bringing the total number of active cases to 283, with three in intensive care. There have been a total of 8,590 cases. Nine have been discharged, bringing the total number of recovered to 8,186. The death toll remains at 121.
- New Zealand has reported two news cases, bringing the total number of active cases to ten after one person recovered. There are a total of 1,515 cases (1,165 cases and 350 probable cases). One person has recovered, bringing the total number of recoveries to 1,483. The death toll remains at 22.
- Singapore has reported 119 new cases, bringing the total to 42,432. In addition, a patient who recovered from COVID-19 died due to heart disease.
- Ukraine has reported 833 new cases and 23 new deaths, bringing the total numbers to 38,074 and 1,035, respectively; a total of 16,956 patients have recovered.
- Tennis player Novak Djokovic and his wife tested positive.

- Boris Johnson leads the UK government's final Downing Street daily briefing. From now on, press briefings will be held whenever there is a significant announcement.
- Doctors have expressed concern that a significant number of COVID-19 patients may be left with the permanent lung condition pulmonary fibrosis as a result of the virus and will need to be monitored for signs of the condition.
- Health officials in Beijing announced that the city's daily testing capacity will be increased to over 300,000 after a number of cases linked to a wholesale market were reported.
- The manager of Tokyo Disneyland revealed that the park will reopen on July 1.
- In South Korea, officials in the city of Daegu announced they would take legal action against the Shincheonji Church of Jesus, claiming that the church contributed significantly to the spread of COVID-19 in the city and failed to implement restrictions when instructed by authorities.
- United Nations Secretary-General António Guterres on International Widow's Day called for countries to work towards dismantling laws that discriminate against women, particularly over inheritance, as they built back from the COVID-19 pandemic.
- The Malaysian Ministry of Education has shortened both mid-year and end-of-the-year holidays to help schools better plan lessons that had been disrupted by the COVID-19 pandemic and lockdown. The mid-term break would be reduced from nine days to five days. The end of the year holidays would be reduced from 42 to 43 days to 14–13 days depending on the state. The Education Ministry confirmed

that the 2020 school year will total 168 days. In response, former Education Minister Maszlee Malik criticised the Ministry for not consulting with teachers and teachers' unions prior to amending the school calendar.

- Zafar Mirza, a health adviser to Prime Minister of Pakistan Imran Khan, announced that authorities had identified 500 coronavirus hotspots around the country which could have some lockdown measures reimposed to contain the spread of the virus.
- The Red Cross announced that it would provide 800,000 face coverings to people in vulnerable categories in Thailand.
- Prime Minister of Egypt Moustafa Madbouly announced that the country's night-time curfew would end on June 27. On the same date, restaurants will be permitted to reopen at a reduced capacity, and places of worship can open for daily prayers.
- The government of Oman announced that malls, factories, and non-essential businesses such as travel agencies and estate agents will be allowed to reopen from June 24. However, a social distance of two metres must be maintained between customers and staff.
- The leaders of the European Union announced that they will meet in Brussels on July 17 to discuss the proposed 500 billion euros economic recovery package.
- The French pharmaceutical company Sanofi stated that it aimed to get approval for its coronavirus vaccine being developed with GlaxoSmithKline in the first half of 2020.
- In Germany, the State Minister of Health in North Rhine-Westphalia Karl-Josef Laumann announced that the districts

of Warendorf and Guetersloh had been placed under lockdown to prevent further transmission of the virus after cases were reported at a meatpacking factory in the region. A report also found that the German economy could shrink by up to 6.5 percent in 2020 due to the coronavirus pandemic.

- In the Russian capital of Moscow, restaurants, nurseries, and leisure facilities have reopened after Mayor of Moscow Sergey Sobyanin announced an easing of coronavirus lockdown restrictions two weeks ago.
- Spanish health authorities announced they will trial a coronavirus tracing app on the island of La Gomera from June 26.
- British Prime Minister Boris Johnson announced the easing of several lockdown restrictions from July 4, including allowing members of two different households to meet inside and replacing the 2-meter social distancing rule with a "1-meter-plus" approach. Most businesses will also reopen, including restaurants, bars, hotels, hairdressers, cinemas, and museums. However, other businesses will remain closed, including gyms, pools, spas, and tattoo parlours. Places of worship will be allowed to reopen, and people may attend religious services. England's Chief Medical Officer Chris Whitty also stated that the virus would likely be spreading in the UK in spring 2021.
- Restaurants in groups, and travel on public transport from July 1. He further stated that football matches will reopen to the public after the summer.
- The United Kingdom's Airport Operators Association revealed that as many as 20,000 jobs could be lost at British

airports due to companies' financial losses during the pandemic.

- The first trials for a potential coronavirus vaccine have begun in South Africa, making them the first trials in the African continent. South African pharmaceutical company Aspen Pharmacare also announced that it could potentially produce 10 million dexamethasone tablets in a month.
- Clinical trials of a potential coronavirus vaccine developed by the University of Oxford and AstraZeneca began in Brazil, involving over 3000 participants in Rio de Janeiro and São Paulo.

24 June

- Malaysia has reported six new cases. There are 244 active cases, bringing the total number to 8,596 cases. 45 more cases have been discharged, bringing the total number of recovered to 8,231. The death toll remains at 121.
- New Zealand has reported one new case, bringing the number of active cases to 11. There are a total of 1,516 cases (1,166 cases and 350 probable cases). The total number of recovered and dead remains at 1,483 and 22 respectively.
- Singapore has reported 191 new cases, bringing the total to 42,623.
- Ukraine sets a new record for daily cases at 940 and reports 16 new deaths. The totals are now 39,014 cases and 1,051 lethal outcomes. Additionally, 17,409 patients have recovered overall.
- Sacramento Kings players Buddy Hield, Alex Len, and Jabari Parker tested positive for the virus.

- Scientists at Imperial College London begin human trials of a COVID-19 vaccine after tests on animals indicate an effective immune response; 300 volunteers will take part in the programme.
- The British Medical Journal publishes an open letter from health leaders in which they call on the government to launch an urgent review to determine whether the UK is prepared for what they describe as the "real risk" of the second wave of COVID-19.
- The UK government publishes new advice for businesses on how to safely reopen their premises on 4 July.
- 170 United Nations Member States and Observers endorsed the United Nations Secretary General's global ceasefire appeal during the COVID crisis.
- The International Monetary Fund, in its latest World Economic Outlook report, warned that the economic recovery from the COVID-19 pandemic was projected to be slower than previously forecast, with growth in 2020 estimated at -4.9 percent, or nearly two percentage points below April projections, indicating a deeper recession and slower recovery.
- The World Health Organization Director-General warned that the world was on track to reach 10 million coronavirus cases within the next week, a “sober reminder” that as research continues into therapeutics and vaccines, maximum efforts were required immediately to suppress transmission and save lives.
- Health authorities in the Australian state of Victoria announced that 1,000 Australian Defence Force personnel

will be deployed to Melbourne to deal with a recent spike in coronavirus cases.

- Authorities in the Chinese capital of Beijing announced that the city's recent outbreak of coronavirus was under control.
- President of the Philippines, Rodrigo Duterte, revealed that the Philippine government was planning a 4.3 trillion peso ($86 billion) budget for 2021 to aid the country's economic recovery from the coronavirus pandemic.
- President of the Maldives Ibrahim Mohamed Solih announced that international tourists from all countries will be allowed to enter the Maldives from July 15.
- Emirates Airlines suspended flights from Pakistan after a number of passengers tested positive for COVID-19.
- Health authorities in Israel reimposed lockdown restrictions in Tiberias and the town of Elad after a rise in cases.
- Qatar Airways announced that daily flights to the Lebanese capital of Beirut would resume from July 1after previously being suspended due to coronavirus concerns.
- Chancellor of Austria Sebastian Kurz advised citizens against all travel to the German state of North Rhine-Westphalia after a surge in cases linked to a meat processing plant there.
- Bulgarian Health Minister Kiril Ananiev announced that Bulgaria's state of emergency will be extended to July 15 due to consistent rises in coronavirus cases.
- Health authorities in Kazakhstan placed the towns of Kokshetau and Stepnogorsk in lockdown by introducing a curfew, blocking access by road, and closing all non-essential venues.

- Prime Minister of the Netherlands Mark Rutte announced a further easing of lockdown restrictions in the country that will see the population allowed to meet, gather outdoors and visit
- Finance Minister of South Africa Tito Mboweni announced that the country's economy is expected to shrink by 7.2 percent in 2020, the largest decrease in ninety years.
- The International Monetary Fund revealed that the global economy is predicted to contract by 4.9 percent as a direct result of the coronavirus pandemic, nearly 2 percent more than what was predicted in April, with economic losses estimated at $12 trillion.
- Apple Inc. announced that seven stores in Houston would be closed due to a rise in coronavirus cases in the US.
- Governor of Washington Jay Inslee announced that it would be mandatory for all residents to wear face coverings in public after a surge in cases.
- Organisers of the New York City Marathon announced that the 2020 event would be cancelled due to the coronavirus pandemic. Governor of New York Andrew Cuomo also released a statement alongside Governor of New Jersey Phil Murphy and Governor of Connecticut Ned Lamont, which stated that anybody arriving from states with high rates of coronavirus would have to undergo a mandatory 14-day quarantine upon arrival as a result of the rising cases.

25 June

- Israel has reported 668 new cases, bringing the total number of cases to 6,000, with 47 in serious condition and 29 on ventilators. A total of 186 have been hospitalized, and 16,007 have recovered.
- Malaysia has reported 4 new cases, bringing the number of active cases to 208, with two in intensive care. There are a total of 8,600 cases. 40 patients have recovered, bringing the total number of recovered to 8,271.
- New Zealand has reported three new cases, bringing the number of active cases to 13. There are a total of 1,519 cases (1,169 confirmed and 350 probable cases). One person recovered, bringing the total number of recoveries to 1,484. The death toll remains 22. All three new cases resulted from overseas travel, with two in Christchurch and one in Rotorua.
- Miami Heat player Derrick Jones Jr. tests positive for the virus.
- Singapore has reported 113 new cases, bringing the total to 42,736.
- Ukraine sets a new record for daily cases at 994 and reports 16 new deaths. The totals are now 40,008 cases and 1,067 lethal outcomes. Additionally, 17,758 patients have recovered overall.
- In a letter to the British Medical Journal, a group of senior health academics expresses their concern that COVID-19 antibody tests for NHS and care staff are being rolled out without "adequate assessment" and will place the health service under unnecessary strain.

- As the UK experiences a short heatwave, Bournemouth, Christchurch, and Poole Council declare a major incident after half a million people travel to the Dorset coast. Professor Chris Whitty, the UK's chief medical officer, warns people to respect social distancing guidelines while enjoying the weather, or the number of COVID-19 cases "will rise again."
- The weekly ONS household survey for 8–21 June estimates that new infections were occurring at a rate of 22,000 per week and notes that the decline seen between mid-May and early June has "levelled off."
- The UK government announces plans to relax rules for England and Wales, allowing pubs and restaurants to utilise outdoor spaces such as terraces, pavements, and car parks. In contrast, outdoor markets and fetes will no longer need planning permission.
- The United Nations Secretary-General launched the 'UN Comprehensive Response to COVID-19', a major policy document to coordinate the United Nations System to "save lives, protect societies, recover better" during and after the pandemic.
- The UN Office on Drugs and Crime (UNODC) released its latest annual report, noting that over 35 million people globally now suffer from drug addiction. The report also analyzes the far-reaching impact of the coronavirus pandemic on global drug markets.
- Health authorities in the US revealed that up to 20 million Americans could have contracted COVID-19 despite official figures suggesting only 2.3 million cases have been recorded.

- Governor of California Gavin Newsom declared a budget emergency after the state revealed it was expecting a $54 billion budget deficit. California's Disneyland also announced that it had been forced to postpone reopening on July 17 due to rising coronavirus cases in California.
- Governor of Texas Greg Abbott stated that authorities had decided to temporarily pause the reopening of businesses in the state as a result of rising coronavirus cases.
- American company Macy's announced that almost 4,000 staff had lost their jobs due to the economic implications of the coronavirus pandemic.
- Australia's national airline Qantas announced that a further 6,000 staff will lose their jobs at the company as the airline struggles to deal with the economic implications of the coronavirus pandemic.
- Indonesia's Ministry of Environment and Forestry announced that protection for the Indonesian rainforest had been scaled back as part of budget cuts caused by the coronavirus pandemic during the season most vulnerable to forest fires.
- Health authorities in the Indian capital of New Delhi announced that all 29 million residents of the city would complete a survey regarding their health, with the aim of identifying as many potential cases of the virus as possible.
- The national airline of Egypt EgyptAir announced that the company would resume domestic and international flights from July.
- Prime Minister of Israel Benjamin Netanyahu stated that a number of Israeli companies would be collaborating with two private companies from the United Arab Emirates on various medical projects, including some linked to coronavirus.

- In France, the Eiffel Tower was reopened to the public with strict hygiene and social distancing measures in place. France's Minister for Youth Affairs and Sports, Roxana Mărăcineanu, also announced that financial assistance for the country's sports industry would be extended to September.
- Shareholders in Germany's national airline Lufthansa announced their support for a 9 billion euro ($10 billion) government payout to protect the company from collapsing amidst the coronavirus pandemic after it was reported that the airline was days away from becoming bankrupt. The agreement will see the German government take a 20 percent share in the company, with the airline undergoing a restructuring programme to cut costs.
- Kazakhstan's Health Minister Eljan Birtanov resigned, citing complications due to coronavirus.
- Prime Minister of Norway Erna Solberg confirmed that Norway will reopen its borders to European countries that meet certain criteria from July 15.
- Authorities in the Greater Lisbon region in Portugal announced that a stay-at-home rule would be reimposed in a total of 19 districts from June 29 due to a rise in coronavirus cases.
- Spanish authorities have extended the country's furlough scheme until September 30 to minimise the economic implications of the pandemic.
- President of Senegal Macky Sall announced he would be self-isolating for two weeks after coming into contact with a person who later tested positive for COVID-19.

26 June

- Indonesia has reported 1,240 new cases and 63 new deaths. The totals are now 51,427 cases and 2,683 deaths.
- Malaysia has reported six new cases, bringing the total to 8,606. There are 200 active cases, with two in intensive care. 23 patients have been discharged, bringing the total number of recovered to 8,294. The death toll remains at 121.
- Mexico has reported 5,441 new cases and 719 new deaths, totalling 208,392 cases and 25,779 deaths.
- New Zealand has reported one new case, bringing the number of active cases to 14. There are 1,520 cases (1,170 confirmed and 350 probable cases). There are 1,484 recoveries and 22 deaths.
- Singapore has reported 219 new cases, bringing the total to 42,955.
- Ukraine sets a new record for daily cases at 1,109 and reports 19 new deaths. The totals are now 41,117 cases and 1,086 lethal outcomes. Additionally, 18,299 patients have recovered overall.
- Prime Minister Boris Johnson warns that the UK could be set back if people continue to ignore social distancing rules as those who visited the south coast the previous day have done.
- Professor Neil Ferguson, a former government scientific adviser, says he does not believe a second national lockdown would be necessary but instead would expect to see "targeted" measures to deal with outbreaks.
- Research published by the University of Oxford's Centre for Evidence-Based Medicine shows that the proportion of COVID hospital patients dying each day in England has

fallen from 6% to 1% between April and June. In terms of numbers, 15,468 people were in hospital in England, of which 899 died (6%) on 8 April, compared to 2,698 hospital patients on 21 June, 30 of which died (1%).

- Intu Properties, an owner of many of the UK's largest shopping centres, goes into administration because of the financial impact of the COVID-19 outbreak.
- The UK government confirms that people returning from certain countries will not be required to quarantine for 14 days when returning to the UK from 6 July. A traffic lights system will be established, allocating colours depending on a country's risk level, with a list of countries to be confirmed at a later date.
- The World Health Organization and partners warned that more than $31 billion would be needed over the next 12 months to develop effective medicines for COVID-19 and make them globally available to all people.
- UNICEF warned in a new report that the number of malnourished children in Yemen could reach 2.4 million by the end of 2020 due to huge shortfalls in humanitarian aid funding amid the coronavirus pandemic.
- The Chinese capital of Beijing partially lifted the coronavirus lockdown in place in districts affected by an outbreak linked to a wholesale market in the city.
- The Secretary-General of ASEAN Lim Jock Hoi announced that the region's economy was predicted to contract for the first time in 22 years after Prime Minister of Vietnam Nguyễn Xuân Phúc warned that the pandemic had "swept away the successes of recent years."

- President of Argentina Alberto Fernández announced that tighter restrictions will be implemented in Buenos Aires in response to a large increase in cases.
- Costa Rica's Health Minister Daniel Salas revealed that the country would reopen its borders to international travellers from certain countries with low transmission rates on August 1. This comes as the World Bank provided a $300 million loan to the Costa Rican government to ease the economic consequences of the pandemic.
- Data suggests that the Mexican economy contracted by 17 percent as a direct result of restrictions imposed during the coronavirus pandemic, making it the largest contraction in the country's history.
- Vice President of the United States Mike Pence announced that sixteen states are experiencing rises in coronavirus cases, sparking concerns over a second wave of the virus. This comes as the number of cases rose by its biggest amount to date yesterday.
- American Airlines announced that flights would resume at full capacity from July 1.
- Governor of Texas Greg Abbott announced that bars will be forced to close, and restaurants will have to reduce capacity as coronavirus cases surge in the state. . The local authorities must also approve outdoor gatherings of more than 100 people.
- The International Monetary Fund approved a loan of $5.2 billion to aid Egypt's recovery from the coronavirus pandemic.
- The Regional Director for Europe from the World Health Organization, Hans Kluge, warned that the continent was at

the risk of a second wave of coronavirus infections after authorities identified 30 countries having seen recent increases.

- Scientists from Spain's University of Barcelona revealed that traces of COVID-19 had been identified in waste water collected in March 2019, which, if confirmed, would raise concerns over the spread of the virus before a public health emergency was confirmed in December. However, authorities stated that it was most likely a contaminated sample.
- Authorities in South Africa announced that casinos and cinemas will be permitted to reopen from June 29.

27 June

- Canada reported 274 new cases, bringing a total of 103,032 cases.
- Malaysia has reported ten new cases, bringing the total to 8,616. There are 187 active cases, with two in intensive care. 14 patients have been discharged, bringing the total number of recovered to 8,307. The death toll remains at 121. As of 25 June, 61,576 Malaysians have returned from overseas, with 610 testings positive for COVID-19.
- New Zealand has reported two new cases, bringing the number of active cases to 16. There are a total of 1,522 cases (1,172 confirmed and 350 probable). There are a total of 1,484 recoveries and 22 deaths.
- Singapore has reported 291 new cases, bringing the total to 43,246. In addition, a patient who had COVID died from height injuries.

- Ukraine has reported 948 new cases and 24 new deaths, bringing the total numbers to 42,065 and 1,110, respectively; a total of 18,701 patients have recovered.
- The U.S. set a record number of cases with 44,732 cases.
- There are now over 10 million coronavirus cases, with over 500,000 deaths.
- Travel companies report that holiday bookings have "exploded" since the UK government announced plans to ease quarantine restrictions on travel abroad. But Scotland says it is yet to decide on the matter. Although the UK government has authority over border control, the Scottish government must be consulted on quarantine in Scotland because health matters in Scotland are devolved to the Scottish government.
- The Red Arrows perform a fly-past over Scarborough for Armed Forces Day; a celebration in the town for the occasion was cancelled because of the COVID-19 outbreak.
- Pakistan's Minister for Science and Technology, Fawad Chaudhry, announced that the country has started producing locally designed ventilators.
- President of Sri Lanka, Gotabaya Rajapaksa, lifted the country's coronavirus lockdown after a sustained drop in the number of cases, with one official stating that there was "no community transmission" in the country.
- Authorities in Egypt lifted some coronavirus restrictions throughout the country, including reopening places of worship, restaurants, gyms, and theatres at a reduced capacity. The country's night curfew was also lifted.

- Supreme Leader of Iran Ali Khamenei warned that the country's economic crisis would be worsened if there were to be the second wave of coronavirus infections in the country.
- The European Union delayed a decision to reopen borders to tourists from outside the Schengen area. Diplomats stated that the changes could come into effect from July 1 at the earliest and that the US, Brazil, and Russia would almost certainly be excluded due to high rates of infection.
- Chancellor of Germany Angela Merkel urged German citizens to be cautious and adhere to restrictions as the country's economy begins to ease out of lockdown.
- The British Government announced an easing of the rule requiring anyone arriving in the country to enter a mandatory 14-day quarantine. Authorities stated that tourists would be allowed to visit countries deemed to have low risks of coronavirus infections, with the full list set to be released next week.
- Brazil's Ministry of Health announced that the country had spent $127 million to produce the coronavirus vaccine developed by AstraZeneca and the University of Oxford.
- Peruvian authorities announced the easing of lockdown restrictions in most areas of the country, including the capital Lima. Banks and supermarkets will be permitted to reopen at a reduced capacity, and people will be required to wear a face-covering and maintain a social distance of one metre. Despite this, the government confirmed that the country's curfew would remain in place and that international borders would remain closed.

28 June

- Data from Johns Hopkins University shows that global cases and deaths have passed 10 million and 500,000, respectively.
- Brazil reported 46,860 new cases and 990 deaths, bringing the totals to 1,274,974 cases and 55,961 deaths.
- Kuwait recorded 551 new coronavirus cases, bringing the country's total to 44,942. 908 people recovered, bringing the total number of recoveries to 35,494. A further 4 deaths were reported.
- Malaysia has reported 18 new cases (four Malaysians and 14 foreigners), bringing the total number to 8,634. There are 195 active cases, with two in intensive care. Ten patients have recovered, bringing the total number of recovered to 8,318. The death toll remains at 121.
- New Zealand has reported four new international travel-related cases bringing the number of active cases to 20, with 1,526 cases (1,176 confirmed and 350 probable), 1,484 recoveries, and 22 deaths.
- Singapore has reported 213 new cases, bringing the total to 43,459.
- Ukraine has reported 917 new cases and 19 new deaths, bringing the total numbers to 42,982 and 1,129, respectively; a total of 18,934 patients have recovered.
- The United Kingdom recorded 901 new cases and 36 deaths, bringing the totals to 311,151 and 43,550, respectively. There were no new fatalities in Scotland for the third consecutive day.

- The United States of America recorded 44,458 cases and 650 new deaths, bringing the country's totals to 2,452,048 and 124,811, respectively.
- The Australian state of Victoria announced that mandatory coronavirus tests for arriving travellers would be introduced after a sharp spike in infections.
- Authorities in China have placed 400,000 under a strict coronavirus lockdown in Anxin County in the state of Hebei after a surge in cases near the capital of Beijing related to a wholesale market, meaning only essential workers will be permitted to leave their homes and that non-residents will not be allowed to enter buildings or communities.
- Singaporean Prime Minister Lee Hsien Loong and Malaysian Prime Minister Muhyiddin Yassin have agreed that their governments will work together to establish a Periodic Commuting Arrangement (PCA), allowing residents from both nations who hold long-term immigration passes for business and work purposes in the other country to periodically return to their home countries for short-term home leave.
- Authorities in South Korea announced that fans will be allowed to attend some sports fixtures at a limited capacity.
- Home Secretary Priti Patel confirms a Sunday Times report that the government is considering imposing a local lockdown on Leicester, which has seen a spike in COVID-19 cases. Of the 2,494 cases reported in the city, 658 (around 25%) occurred in the two weeks preceding 16 June.
- President of Iran Hassan Rouhani announced that wearing face masks will be mandatory in some parts of the country from next week. Rouhani further stated that Iran was facing

the "most difficult year" in the country's history as a result of the coronavirus pandemic and the United States sanctions against Iran.

- . In July, the Irish government has stated that it will maintain a 14-day mandatory quarantine for British tourists.
- Authorities in the Swiss city of Zürich announced that 300 people have been put in a mandatory quarantine following a surge in cases linked to a nightclub in the city.
- The Turkish Interior Ministry has imposed a nationwide daytime curfew during university entrance exam season to prevent large gatherings.
- British Home Secretary Priti Patel announced that the city of Leicester might be placed in a regional lockdown after it was revealed that 25 percent of the city's coronavirus cases had been reported in the last two weeks. Such a measure would be the first of its kind in the UK.
- Data gathered by Johns Hopkins University in the United States suggests that the global number of deaths from COVID-19 has surpassed 500,000, with over 10 million people having been infected.
- St. Patrick's Cathedral in New York City reopened for Sunday Mass with a reduced capacity and strict social distancing in place.

29 June

- Malaysia has reported three new cases, bringing the total number to 8,637. There are 182 active cases. 16 people have recovered, bringing the total number of recovered to 8,334. The death toll remains at 121.
- New Zealand has reported two new international travel-related cases, bringing the number of active cases to 22, with a total number of 1,528 cases (1,178 confirmed and 350 probable), 1,484 recoveries, and 22 deaths.
- Singapore has reported 202 new cases, bringing the total to 43,661.
- Ukraine has reported 646 new cases and 18 new deaths, bringing the total numbers to 43,628 and 1,147, respectively; a total of 19,027 patients have recovered.
- Following a spike in COVID-19 cases in Leicester, Health Secretary Matt Hancock announces the reintroduction of stricter lockdown measures for the city, including the closure of non-essential retailers from the following day and the closure of schools from 2 July. People in Leicester are advised to stay at home as much as possible, while it is recommended that all but essential travel to, from, and within the city should be avoided. Of the 2,987 positive cases in Leicester since the pandemic began, 866 (29%) were reported in the two weeks preceding 23 June, while Hancock says Leicester accounted for "10% of all positive cases in the country over the past week". Sir Peter Soulsby, the Mayor of Leicester, has criticises a lack of communication between the UK government and Leicester City Council, which he describes as "intensely frustrating."

- The UK government announces that mandatory MOT tests will be reintroduced from 1 August.
- The analysis produced by the BBC indicated that the UK had been the worst hit of the G7 countries in terms of COVID-19, while England is the worst-hit nation of Europe, just ahead of Spain.
- The Greek Government extends its ban on flights from the UK until 15 July.
- The England and Wales Cricket Board confirms that the 2020 County Championship season will begin on 1 August.
- Director-General of the World Health Organization Tedros Adhanom has said that a team from the World Health Organization will be sent to China in the coming weeks to investigate the origins of the COVID-19 after pressure from the international community.
- New Zealand Health Minister David Clark has announced that the New Zealand Government will be investing NZ$150 million in personal protective equipment and requiring returnees in isolation facilities to wear face masks.
- The minister of North Rhine-Westphalia in Germany, Armin Laschet, extended the lockdown restrictions in the district of Guetersloh by a further week, which would see non-essential businesses and leisure facilities remain closed.
- President of Kazakhstan Kassym-Jomart Tokayev has reportedly instructed the Kazakh government to prepare a package of coronavirus restrictions after a sustained increase of cases and deaths in the country. He ordered hospital capacity to be increased by 50 percent within a month and the construction of mobile testing facilities.

- President of Turkey, Recep Tayyip Erdoğan, extended the country's wage support scheme and financial aid to lower-income households to deal with the economic consequences of the coronavirus pandemic.
- British Health Secretary Matt Hancock announced that the city of Leicester had been placed in the UK's first local lockdown after 25 percent of the city's cases were reported in the last two weeks. Under the new restrictions, non-essential businesses have been told to close, and most schools will close from July 2. Travel to and from the city was also strongly discouraged.
- Authorities in Thailand announced that international flights to and from the country will resume from July 1 and that pubs and bars will be permitted to reopen on the same date.
- The government of Bahrain announced that it would pay 50 percent of wages for private firm employees damaged by the coronavirus pandemic.
- Authorities in Qatar have revealed that more coronavirus restrictions will be eased from July 1, including reopening restaurants, beaches, and offices at 50 percent capacity. Gatherings of up to five people will also be permitted.
- In the United Arab Emirates, it was announced that all government employees will return to work from July 5, although social distancing measures would remain in place.
- Kenya's tourism ministry revealed that the country had lost over $750 million in tourism revenues as a direct result of coronavirus restrictions.
- Nigerian authorities have stated that travel between states will be allowed from July 1 and that students due to graduate in the summer will return to school to prepare for exams.

- Governor of São Paulo João Doria announced that he is expecting approval from Brazil's federal regulator to trial a possible COVID-19 vaccine developed by the Chinese company Sinovac Biotech. This comes as the World Health Organization urged federal and state authorities to work more closely to combat the pandemic in Brazil.
- Canadian Prime Minister Justin Trudeau urged Canadians to be cautious as the country slowly reopens its economy.
- Governor of New York Andrew Cuomo urged Donald Trump to sign an executive order making it mandatory to wear face coverings in public. Theatres in New York's Broadway extended their closures to January 2021.
- Los Angeles County announced that beaches will be closed during the July 4 Independence Day holiday weekend after continued daily increases in cases.

30 June

- Malaysia has reported two new cases, bringing the total number to 8,639. There are 164 active cases. 20 people were discharged, bringing the total number of recovered to 8,354. The death toll remains at 121.
- New Zealand has reported no new cases, keeping the number of active cases at 22, with a total number of 1,528 cases (1,178 confirmed and 350 probable), 1,484 recoveries, and 22 deaths.
- Singapore has reported 246 new cases, bringing the total to 43,907.
- Ukraine has reported 706 new cases and 12 new deaths, bringing the total numbers to 44,334 and 1,159, respectively; a total of 19,115 patients have recovered.

- Worldwide, cases are growing at the rate of about 1 to 2 percent per day. Between 100,000 and 200,000 new cases are being detected every day. This number is higher than the number of recoveries every day, in the range of 80,000 to 130,000.
- As Leicester begins at least two weeks of re-tightened lockdown restrictions, a list of other areas where COVID-19 cases are rising is published, though the increases are much smaller than Leicester.
- Prime Minister Boris Johnson sets out a £5bn post-coronavirus recovery plan for the UK that will see the home building and improvements to infrastructure, describing it as a "new deal."
- Figures from the Office for National Statistics have indicated that the number of deaths in the week up to 19 June fell below thfive-year average for the first time since March.
- Rented motorized scooters are to be permitted on UK roads from 4 July in a bid to ease pressure on public transport.
- EasyJet begins the consultation process for plans to close three of its UK bases.
- Reactions and measures at the United Nations
- The United Nations Secretary-General called on the world to increase “financial, humanitarian and political commitments” to help end nearly a decade of major conflict and suffering in Syria in a message to the fourth Brussels Donor Conference.
- On Social Media Day, the United Nations launched its Verified initiative, which calls on people globally to pause before sharing to help stop the viral spread of COVID-19 misinformation.

- Director-General of the International Labour Organization (ILO) Guy Ryder, commenting on new ILO data showing that working hours fell 14 percent during the second quarter of 2020, stated that the impact of the COVID-19 crisis on jobs had been much worse than initially expected, as he appealed to governments, workers and employers to agree on a sustainable economic recovery plan to reduce the inequalities revealed by the pandemic.
- Canadian authorities extended the country's foreign travel ban to July 31 and the mandatory 14-day for all arriving travellers, including citizens, to August 31 to attempt to slow the spread of coronavirus.
- In the United States, director of the National Institute of Allergy and Infectious Diseases Anthony Fauci warned that the US could say as many as 100,000 new cases of coronavirus a day if people do not adhere to public health recommendations.
- Governor of Arizona Doug Ducey ordered bars, gyms, cinemas, and some other non-essential businesses to close for thirty days after increasing cases of COVID-19. Events with more than fifty people will also be banned.
- Governor of New York Andrew Cuomo added a further eight states to New York's mandatory 14-day quarantine for arriving travellers. The additional states were named California, Georgia, Iowa, Idaho, Louisiana, Mississippi, Nevada, and Tennessee.
- Victorian Premier Daniel Andrews has announced that a lockdown will be re-imposed on ten postcodes in Melbourne for two weeks from 11:59 pm on 1 July in response to a spike of new cases in the city.

- The European Union revealed the 14 countries from which non-essential travel can resume from July. The countries deemed safe were listed as Algeria, Australia, Canada, Georgia, Japan, Montenegro, Morocco, New Zealand, Rwanda, Serbia, South Korea, Thailand, Tunisia, and Uruguay. China will also be included if the government allows travellers from Europe to enter without a mandatory quarantine.
- The Dutch-British company Royal Dutch Shell warned that the value of the company's assets could be cut by $22 billion due to a fall in global oil prices during the coronavirus crisis.
- Spain's Institute of National Statistics revealed that the country's GDP contracted by 5.2 percent in the first three months of the year, the largest decrease in fifty years.
- The government of Uzbekistan has imposed a curfew in the capital city of Tashkent and surrounding areas after a large increase in coronavirus cases. Under new restrictions announced by the government, shopping centres will be required to close at the weekend, and people will be unable to leave their homes during the night.

Pandemic Chronology July 2020

1 July

- Malaysia has reported only one imported case, bringing the number of active cases to 144, with a total of 8,640 cases. 21 patients have recovered, bringing the total to 8,375. The death toll remains at 121.
- New Zealand has reported no new cases, keeping the number of active cases at 22, with a total number of 1,528 cases (1,178 confirmed and 350 probable), 1,484 recoveries, and 22 deaths. One case remains in hospital.
- Singapore has reported 215 new cases, bringing the total to 44,122.
- Ukraine has reported 664 new cases and 14 new deaths, bringing the total numbers to 44,998 and 1,173, respectively; a total of 19,548 patients have recovered.
- Over two days, 12,000 job losses have been announced in the retail and aviation industry as a result of the economic impact of the COVID-19 outbreak.
- Conservative MP Giles Watling warned of the impact on theatres if they have to cancel the pantomime season; his comments come after several theatres announced plans to cancel pantomimes over the coming winter season.
- The United Nations Security Council passed resolution S/RES/2532: 'Maintenance of international peace and security," demanding a global ceasefire. The United Nations Secretary-General announced that unless the world acts immediately, with "bold and creative" solutions, the COVID-19 pandemic and accompanying global recession would trigger "years of depressed and disrupted economic growth".

The Director-General of the World Health Organization stated that some nations battling the COVID-19 pandemic which had been taking a "fragmented approach" to suppressing the deadly virus "face a long, hard road ahead."

- United States Secretary of Health and Human Services Alex Azar announced that the American government had purchased nearly all of the next three months' estimated production of the only licensed COVID-19 therapeutic, remdesivir, from the biopharmaceutical company Gilead Sciences for use in American hospitals, prompting both domestic and international criticism.
- California Governor Gavin Newsom ordered the closure of most indoor businesses in 19 counties.
- Mayor of New York City Bill de Blasio delayed the planned resumption of indoor dining at restaurants in the city over concerns of a possible rise in infections.
- Google announced that the company's offices in the US would remain closed until 7 September after initially being scheduled to reopen on 6 July. The reopening was postponed in response to the surge in coronavirus cases in the country.
- Health authorities in the Australian state of Victoria announced that a stage-three lockdown will be enforced in 36 suburbs north of Melbourne for a month from midnight on 2 July after a recent surge in cases in the area, prompting concerns over a possible second wave of infections. Under the new restrictions, residents will only be allowed to leave their homes for essential reasons, with Premier of Victoria Daniel Andrews warning that tighter restrictions could be brought in if the situation does not improve.

- In Japan, Tokyo Disneyland and Tokyo DisneySea reopened to the public after closing at the peak of the COVID-19 pandemic. Visitors to the attractions must maintain a social distance, book any admission tickets in advance and undergo mandatory temperature checks on arrival, with the number of entrants at a reduced capacity.
- North Korea's Ministry of Public Health has reopened its schools and made it mandatory to wearface-covering in public spaces. The country's ban on large gatherings was also maintained.
- Zimbabwe's Minister of Media, Information, and Publicity Monica Mutsvangwa announced that national parks and wildlife centres will be allowed to reopen and that restaurants will be able to resume indoor dining.
- The national carrier of Egypt EgyptAir resumed operations from Cairo International Airport, with airports reopening to international tourists across the country. Museums and landmarks, including the Giza pyramid complex.
- Israel's national airline El Al revealed that the company had a steep decline in revenue in the first quarter, forcing it to reduce the workforce and fleet of aircraft. Bosses are reportedly requesting state-backed loans to ensure the company's survival.
- Beirut-Rafic Hariri International Airport in the Lebanese capital of Beirut reopened at ten per cent capacity to encourage tourism in the country after the coronavirus pandemic.
- The Palestinian National Authority announced that a five-day lockdown will be imposed in the West Bank after an increase in coronavirus cases.

- The Qatari government began a partial reopening of restaurants, beaches, parks, and places of worship.
- Authorities in the United Arab Emirates stated that residents cannot travel abroad for non-essential purposes yet, and that all foreign travel still requires a permit.
- Austrian Foreign Affairs Minister Alexander Schallenberg warned citizens not to travel to six countries in the Balkans that are not part of the European Union. The six countries were later revealed to be Albania, Bosnia & Herzegovina, Kosovo, Montenegro, North Macedonia, and Serbia.
- Belgium moved into phase 4 of the country's plan to ease coronavirus lockdown restrictions, with cinemas, casinos, and concert halls reopening and 'social bubble' sizes expanding from ten to fifteen people.
- The European Union reopened borders to travellers from fifteen countries deemed to be low-risk for coronavirus transmission.
- European airline manufacturing company Airbus announced it would be cutting 15,000 jobs due to the impact of the COVID-19 pandemic on aviation, with most jobs being lost in the UK, Germany, and Spain.
- Greek authorities reopened the country's borders to international travellers from some countries, with airports and ports reopening across the country.
- The border between Portugal and Spain was officially reopened by President of Portugal Marcelo Rebelo de Sousa and King Felipe VI of Spain after being closed for more than three months to prevent the spread of coronavirus between the two countries.

- The Swiss Federal Councillor for Home Affairs, Alain Berset, announced that a 10-day mandatory quarantine will be enforced on all travellers arriving from countries deemed high-risk from 6 July, in line with the measures introduced by the European Union.
- Malaysian Education Minister Mohd Radzi Md Jidin has announced that schools for other students will reopen in two stages from 15 July. Secondary school pupils, senior primary pupils, and removed class students will return on 15 July, while junior primary pupils will return on 22 July.
- In Thailand, schools and leisure venues such as restaurants reopened with strict social distancing rules and temperature checks in place.

2 July

- Brazil has reported 1,038 new deaths, taking the country's total to 60,632.
- France has reported 14 new deaths, taking the total to 29,875. The number of hospitalised cases decreased by 188 to 8,148, and the total number of people in intensive care fell by 9 to 573.
- Malaysia has reported three new cases, bringing the total number to 8,643 cases with 85 active cases. 62 have recovered, bringing the number of recovered to 8,437. The death toll remains at 121.
- New Zealand has reported two new cases, bringing the total number to 1,530 cases (1,180 confirmed and 350 probable). Six people have recovered, bringing the number of active cases down to 18 and the total number of recoveries to 1,490. The death toll remains at 22.

- Serbia reported 359 new cases and 6 new deaths, bringing the totals to 15,195 and 287, respectively. There are currently 1,996 active cases with 81 patients in intensive care.
- Singapore has reported 188 new cases, bringing the total to 44,310. 418 have recovered, bringing the total number of recovered to 39,429.
- Ukraine has reported 889 new cases and 12 new deaths, bringing the total numbers to 45,887 and 1,185, respectively; a total of 20,053 patients have recovered.
- The United Kingdom reported 89 new deaths, taking the country's official total to 43,995, although estimates place the true number closer to 55,000.
- The United States has reported 50,700 new cases, the highest daily number of new infections recorded so far. The total is over 2.73 million.
- Casual Dining Group, the owner of Café Rouge and Bella Italia, goes into administration with the loss of 1,900 of the 6,000 staff employed by the outlets. At the same time, Airbus announces the loss of 2,730 jobs at two UK factories.
- The weekly ONS household survey for 14–27 June estimates that new infections were occurring in England at a rate of 25,000 per week, a slight increase from their previous report. Blood samples show around 6% of people have antibodies.
- The Secretary-General informed the Security Council that the COVID-19 pandemic was “profoundly affecting” global peace and security across the globe, and he urged it to employ its collective influence to mitigate the protections crisis facing millions of vulnerable people, including those

affected by conflicts. The UN Department of Economic and Social Affairs urged countries' governments to do more support young entrepreneurs in the face of the pandemic as part of a sustainable recovery.

- Hungarian Prime Minister Viktor Orbán announced that countries outside of the European Union, except for Serbia, will not be added to the government's list of safe countries.
- President of Kazakhstan Kassym-Jomart Tokayev introduced a second coronavirus lockdown in the country from 5 July after a rise in infections. Under the new restrictions, non-essential businesses have been forced to close, and travel between provinces has been limited. However, restaurants will be able to remain open for outdoor dining, and people will be allowed to leave their homes.
- Spanish Prime Minister Pedro Sánchez pledged 9 billion euros of emergency funding for the autonomous communities of Spain to improve the country's regional health services and suggested possible tax rises to strengthen the country's economy.
- Authorities in Switzerland revealed that travellers from 29 countries, including the US, Brazil, and Sweden, will have to enter a mandatory 14-day quarantine upon arrival in the country from 6 July to prevent the spread of coronavirus.
- British Secretary of State for Education Gavin Williamson revealed the British government's plans to reopen schools at full capacity in September. It was announced that children will only be able to mix with their own year group with no large events and regular hand-washing. Williamson further stated that staff and students were not expected to wear face masks and that parents would be fined for refusing to send their child to school; pupils showing any symptoms of

COVID-19 must not go to school, and schools reporting any cases would have to be closed.

- British Prime Minister Boris Johnson announced an easing of the country's mandatory 14-day quarantine for anybody arriving from abroad. Countries will be placed in a traffic-light system, whereby travellers from countries in the green and orange "low-risk" categories will not have to self-isolate when arriving in the UK.
- First Minister of Scotland Nicola Sturgeon announced that it will be mandatory to wear face masks in shops from 10 July. Children from different households would no longer need to maintain a social distance when outside.
- King Salman of Saudi Arabia extended various government schemes to support private sector businesses and investors through the economic consequences of the coronavirus pandemic.
- The national airline of the United Arab Emirates Emirates revealed that almost 650,000 refunds had been processed during the coronavirus pandemic, resulting in losses of over $500 million, with the company expecting a further 500,000 refunds to be processed in the next two months.
- New Zealand Health Minister David Clark resigns from his portfolio, stating that "he had become a distraction in the Government's ongoing response to the COVID-19 pandemic in New Zealand and health reforms.
- Cuba eased lockdown restrictions in the capital city Havana, as the remainder of the country moved from phase two to phase three. Under the new restrictions in Havana, public transport resumed, and beaches reopened, although the

government maintained strict social distancing rules and the wearing of face masks.

- The African Union revealed that the African continent had lost $55 billion in travel and tourism revenue during the coronavirus pandemic. The Union's Infrastructure and Energy Committee warned that some African airlines might not survive the economic consequences of the pandemic.
- The coronavirus lockdown imposed in Nigeria's Kano State was lifted.

3 July

- Brazil has reported 37,923 new cases, bringing the total to over 1.5 million. A further 1,091 deaths were recorded, bringing that total to 64,265.
- France has reported 18 new deaths, taking the total to 29,893. It was also reported that the number of people in intensive care fell by 13 to 560.
- India has reported a daily record of 20,903 new cases, bringing the country's total to 625,544. 379 deaths were also recorded, taking the total death toll to 18,213.
- Iran has reported 154 new deaths, taking the country's total to 11,260. The total number of cases was confirmed to stand at 235,429.
- Japan reported 124 new cases in the capital Tokyo, with 70 percent of the infected below the age of forty.
- Malaysia has reported five new cases (three imported and two community transmissions), with the number of active cases being 81 and the total number being 8,648 cases. Nine people have recovered, bringing the number of recovered to 8,446. The death toll remains at 121.

- New Zealand has reported no new cases, with the number of active cases remaining 18 and the total number remaining 1,530 (1,180 confirmed and 350 probable). There have been a total of 1,490 recoveries and 22 deaths.
- Saudi Arabia has reported 4,193 new cases, taking the country's total past 200,000 to 201,801. 1,802 deaths were also reported, with over 140,000 having recovered from the virus.
- Singapore has reported 169 new cases, bringing the total to 44,479. 340 have recovered, bringing the total number of recoveries to 39,769. The death toll remains at 26.
- Spain has reported 17 new deaths in the last 24 hours.
- South Korea has reported 63 new cases, bringing the total to 12,967. The death toll remained at 282.
- Ukraine has reported 876 new cases and 27 new deaths, bringing the total numbers to 46,763 and 1,212, respectively; a total of 20,558 patients have recovered.
- The United Kingdom has reported 137 new deaths, bringing the confirmed total to 44,131, with 544 people testing positive for coronavirus.
- The United States reported 57,683 new cases, the highest daily increase so far, bringing the total number of cases to 2,793,022. A further 728 deaths were also reported, bringing the death toll to 129,405.
- The UK government published a list of 59 countries for which quarantine will not apply when arriving in England as from 10 July. They include Greece, France, Belgium, and Spain, but Portugal and the United States are among those not on the list. These changes do not apply to Scotland, Wales, or

Northern Ireland, where quarantine restrictions remain in place for all arrivals from outside the UK.

- The UK government rushed The Health Protection (Coronavirus, Restrictions) (Leicester) Regulations 2020 through parliament to give police the powers to enforce lockdown restrictions in Leicester as from 4 July.
- UNESCO senior official stated that increased pillaging of endangered World Heritage Sites during COVID-19 lockdowns will likely result in a large number of stolen artifacts appearing online.
- The European Commissioner for Health and Food Safety Stella Kyriakidou announced that the European Commission had approved the use of remdesivir to treat severe cases of coronavirus, the first such drug approved by the European Union.
- In France, the Cour de Justice de la République, a court specialising in government misconduct, announced that an inquiry into the actions of several government ministers' handling of the coronavirus pandemic will be opened, including former Prime Minister Edouard Philippe, former Health Minister Agnès Buzyn and current Health Minister Olivier Véran. The court revealed that all three were accused of "failing to fight a disaster."
- French national airline Air France revealed plans to cut over 7,500 jobs after reportedly losing 15 million euros a day at the height of the coronavirus pandemic.
- The Akim of East Kazakhstan Region Daniyal Akhmetov will impose a full lockdown on the cities of Oskemen and Semey from 5 July due to rising coronavirus cases.

- The Portuguese Ministry of Planning and Infrastructure revealed that the Portuguese government had reached an agreement with shareholders in Portugal's national airline TAP Air to take a controlling stake in an attempt to prevent the company from collapsing due to the economic consequences of the pandemic.
- Serbian President Aleksandar Vučić announced that a state of emergency will be reimposed in the capital city of Belgrade after a surge in coronavirus cases. Under the new restrictions, it will be mandatory to wear face masks in public, and there will be a limit on the size of both indoor and outdoor gatherings.
- The British Government announced that travellers arriving from several countries and territories will not be required to self-isolate for 14 days, including Ireland, the Channel Islands, the Isle of Man, and several European Union countries, Turkey, all British Overseas Territories, Australia, New Zealand, Fiji, Vietnam, South Korea, French Polynesia, and New Caledonia. It was also revealed that the British government was discussing the possibility of joining the EU's plan to secure supplies of a potential coronavirus vaccine.
- According to government data, Japan's Government Pension Investment Fund recorded losses of $77 billion in the most recent fiscal year, the largest decrease since the 2008 financial crisis, which was directly attributed to the coronavirus pandemic.
- Brazilian President Jair Bolsonaro vetoed a law requiring people to wear face masks in shops, schools, and places of worship, stating that such a law could lead to violation of property rights.

- Mayor of Miami-Dade County Carlos A. Giménez imposed an indefinite curfew overnight for the Independence Day holiday weekend. Giménez also delayed the scheduled reopening of entertainment venues, including theatres and casinos, due to a spike in cases in Florida.
- Governor of Texas Greg Abbott introduced legislation making it mandatory to wear a face mask in public due to rising cases of coronavirus in Texas, with fines of up to $250 for those who are caught not wearing a mask.
- Malaysian Minister of Health Adham Baba announced that both Malaysian citizens and foreign nationals traveling to Malaysia would be required to pay fees while undergoing COVID-19 tests.

4 July

- Australia has reported 108 new cases in the state of Victoria, the biggest daily increase since March.
- Azerbaijan has reported 534 new cases, bringing the total to 19,801. The death toll rose to 241, and the number of recoveries was reported to be at almost 11,300.
- Brazil has recorded 37,923
- India has reported a new daily record of 22,772 cases, bringing the total to 648,315. A further 442 deaths were reported, bringing the total death toll thus far to 18,655.
- Malaysia has reported ten new cases, bringing the total to 8,658. There are 76 active cases, with two requiring respiratory support. 15 patients have recovered, bringing the total number of recovered to 8,461. The death toll remains at 121.

- New Zealand has reported no new cases, with the number of active cases at 18 and the total number at 1,530 cases (1,180 confirmed and 350 probable). There have been a total of 1,490 recoveries and 22 deaths.
- Russia has reported 6,632 new cases and 168 new deaths, bringing the totals to 674,515 and 10,027, respectively.
- Singapore has reported 185 new cases, bringing the total to 44,664.
- South Africa has reported 9,064 new cases, the highest daily total so far, with more than 177,000 cases now confirmed in the country.
- South Korea has reported 63 new cases, taking the total to 13,030. The death toll remained at 283.
- Ukraine has reported 914 new cases and 15 new deaths, bringing the total numbers to 47,677 and 1,227, respectively; a total of 21,155 patients have recovered.
- The Health Protection (Coronavirus, Restrictions) (No. 2) (England) Regulations 2020 came into force in England, replacing and relaxing the previous Lockdown Regulations (SI 350) and giving the Secretary of State powers to make declarations restricting access to public outdoor places. Leicester was excluded from the relaxations due to its high rate of COVID-19, with more stringent regulations in force.
- The COVID Symptom Study reports that the two-week average number of new daily cases for the two weeks to 4 July 2020 was no lower than for the previous week; rates of new COVID cases were no longer declining.
- After Brexit Party leader Nigel Farage posted a picture of himself in a pub on Twitter a fortnight after attending a rally in support of US President Donald Trump in the United

States, Ed Davey, the acting leader of the Liberal Democrats, wrote to Kent Police asking them to investigate whether Farage had breached lockdown restrictions. On the same day, Prime Minister Boris Johnson's father, Stanley, had to defend a trip to Greece, which critics say broke restrictions.

- Augusto Santos Silva, the Foreign minister of Portugal, criticised the UK's decision to exclude his country from the list of countries from where travellers do not have to quarantine when returning to the UK as "absurd."
- The National Gallery, set to be the first museum to reopen to the public on 8 July, gave a preview to the media of its new safety measures.
- The UK held a minute's silence to remember those who had died of COVID-19.
- The World Health Organization announced that it would be stopping trials of the antimalarial drug hydroxychloroquine to treat COVID-19 after they failed to reduce the mortality rate amongst hospitalised patients.
- Director of the Louvre museum in Paris Jean-Luc Martinez announced that the popular tourist attraction would reopen to the public from 6 July with strict social distancing rules in place and some areas of the museum remaining closed to visitors. All visitors will be required to book tickets in advance and wear a face mask.
- Greek health authorities announced an extension to coronavirus lockdowns in the country's migrant camps due to concerns over the spread of the virus, despite some international criticism that the government has extended the restrictions to limit the movement of migrants.

- Catalan Health Minister Alba Vergés announced that a local coronavirus lockdown will be enforced in the province of Lleida, affecting 200,000 people due to an outbreak of COVID-19 cases. Under the new restrictions, movement in and out of the area will be heavily restricted by police checkpoints. The capital of the autonomous community of Catalonia, Barcelona, reopened the Sagrada Familia to essential workers and their families as part of an easing of lockdown restrictions there.
- In England, non-essential businesses, including pubs, cinemas, hairdressers, places of worship, and tourist attractions, reopened to the public. Some controversy was generated over the British Government's decision to reopen pubs on a Saturday, with the day being referred to by the media as 'Super Saturday,' sparking concerns over potential violence and breaches of restrictions.
- Iranian President Hassan Rouhani stated that people caught not wearing a face mask in public will be denied access to state services. Employers who fail to follow government guidelines regarding the safety of their workplaces could have their business closed for a week.
- Authorities in Jordan began issuing all arriving travellers with electronic wristbands to enforce the country's coronavirus quarantine rules. All arriving travellers must self-isolate for 14 days at a hotel on the Dead Sea, followed by a further 14-day quarantine at home.
- Data from the Central Bank of Tunisia shows that revenue from the country's tourism industry decreased by 47 per cent in the first half of the year, as a direct consequence of the COVID-19 pandemic.

- Governor of Tokyo Yuriko Koike asked residents not to travel beyond the city's borders to prevent the spread of coronavirus after Tokyo recorded over 100 new cases for the third consecutive day.
- Authorities in Mexico announced that additional health checkpoints will be installed along the Mexico-United States border over concerns of a potential surge of border crossings during the Independence Day holiday weekend in the United States.
- United States President Donald Trump extended the country's Paycheck Protection Program relief fund for businesses to 8 August.
- The cabinet of eSwatini was placed in quarantine after Transport Minister Ndlaluhlaza Ndwandwe tested positive for COVID-19 on Tuesday. Restaurants and casinos reopened in South Africa at a reduced capacity with strict social distancing rules in place.

5 July

- Malaysia has reported five new cases, with the number of active cases at 77 and the total number at 8,663. Four patients have recovered, bringing the total number of recovered to 8,465. The death toll remains at 121.
- New Zealand has reported three new cases, with the number of active cases at 21 and the total number at 1,533 cases (1,183 confirmed and 340 probable). There have been a total of 1,490 recoveries and 22 deaths.
- Singapore has reported 136 new cases, bringing the total to 44,800. 324 have been discharged as of Sunday, bringing the total number of recoveries to 40,441.

- Ukraine has reported 823 new cases and 22 new deaths, bringing the total numbers to 48,500 and 1,249, respectively; a total of 21,376 patients have recovered.
- The UK stages a national round of applause to mark the 72nd anniversary of the founding of the National Health Service; a Supermarine Spitfire flypast over several hospitals in the East of England also takes place to mark the occasion.
- Managers of India's Taj Mahal tourist attraction in Agra announced that it will remain closed for the foreseeable future due to public health concerns.
- Authorities in Greece announced that the country's border will be closed to Serbian travellers until 15 July after the country declared a state of emergency on 3 July in response to rising coronavirus cases.
- Irish Transport Minister Eamon Ryan stated that the country will ease foreign travel restrictions from 20 July. Similar to measures adopted by the United Kingdom, travellers arriving from countries deemed to be low-risk will be exempt from quarantine for 14 days upon the arrival.
- The Government of Kazakhstan announced a further tightening of lockdown restrictions in the country due to a surge in cases. Under the new restrictions, malls, salons, and leisure facilities have been ordered to close for two weeks.
- The British Government revealed an investment of over £1.5 billion to support the country's arts industry, with emergency grants available for theatres, museums, galleries, and cinemas.

- President of the State of Palestine Mahmoud Abbas declared a state of emergency across Palestine for thirty days, with residents only permitted to leave their homes for essential reasons.
- Non-essential American diplomats have been leaving Saudi Arabia due to the surging coronavirus cases in the country.
- President of Chile Sebastián Piñera revealed an economic stimulus package of $1.5 billion to assist the country's struggling economy during the pandemic. The measures available include access to zero-interest loans and subsidised rent.
- President of El Salvador Nayib Bukele delayed moving the country into the second phase of lifting coronavirus lockdown restrictions to 21 July, blaming the increasing number of cases.
- Authorities in Ghana announced that President Nana Akufo-Addo will enter a 14-day self-isolation after coming into contact with an individual who later tested positive for COVID-19.
- Health officials in Madagascar placed the region of Analamanga, containing the capital city of Antananarivo, into a second coronavirus lockdown due to a sudden spike in infections. Under the new restrictions, schools and places of worship have been ordered to close. All non-essential travel has been banned until at least 20 July, with gatherings of more than fifty individuals also prohibited.
- Newly elected President of Malawi Lazarus Chakwera announced that his inauguration ceremony and the country's Independence Day celebrations would be scaled back due to public health concerns.

6 July

- The Australian state of Victoria has reported 127 cases, the biggest overnight spike in Australia since the pandemic began. Australia also recorded two deaths, bringing the death toll to 106.
- Fiji reported the country's first case in 78 days in a tourist returning from India.
- France reported 27 new deaths, taking the total to 29,920. The number of patients in intensive care was recorded to have fallen by 12 to 548.
- India reported 24,428 new cases, bringing the country's total to 697,413.
- Indonesia reported 1,209 new cases and 70 new deaths, bringing the totals to 64,958 and 3,241, respectively.
- Malaysia has reported five new cases, bringing the number of active cases to 77 and the total number to 8,668. 11 cases have been discharged, bringing the total number of recovered to 8,476.
- New Zealand has reported one new case, bringing the number of active cases to 22 and the total number to 1,534 cases (1,184 confirmed and 350 probable). There have been a total of 1,490 recoveries and 22 deaths.
- Pakistan reported 3,344 new cases, including Health Secretary Zafar Mirza, bringing the total to 231,818. 50 new deaths were also reported, bringing that total to 4,844.
- Qatar reported 546 new cases and 5 new deaths, bringing the totals to 100,345 and 133, respectively.
- Singapore has reported 183 new cases, bringing the total to 44,983.

- Ukraine has reported 543 new cases and 13 new deaths, bringing the total numbers to 49,043 and 1,262, respectively; a total of 21,703 patients have recovered.
- The United Kingdom reported 16 new deaths, the lowest figure since 16 March, bringing the total to 44,236. No new deaths were reported in Scotland, Wales, or Northern Ireland.
- The United States passed 130,000 deaths to record a total of 130,007. It was also reported that the total number of cases had reached 2,888,729.
- Vietnam reported 14 imported cases, bringing the country's total number of cases to 369. No further deaths have been reported, with 90% of cases having recovered.
- The UK government announces grants and loans of £1.57bn to support theatres, galleries, museums, and other cultural venues affected by the COVID-19 outbreak.
- As concerns about increasing unemployment grow, the UK government announces a £111m scheme to help firms in England provide an extra 30,000 trainee places; £21m will be provided to fund similar schemes in Scotland, Wales, and Northern Ireland.
- Sandwich retailer Pret a Manger announces plans to close 30 outlets with the loss of 1,000 jobs.
- The BBC's Panorama programme reports that scientific research has suggested the COVID-19 outbreak could result in several thousand extra cancer deaths due to delayed diagnosis and treatment, with estimates being between 7,000 and 35,000.
- No new deaths are reported for Wales for the most recent 24-hour period.

- The Victorian Premier Daniel Andrews and New South Wales Premier Gladys Berejiklian have closed the border between their states for the first time since the Spanish flu pandemic of 1918–1919 in response to a spike of cases in Victoria, which recorded 127 cases overnight.
- Governor of São Paulo João Doria stated that the Brazilian government will start the third phase of clinical trials of a potential vaccine for COVID-19 developed by Chinese biopharmaceutical company Sinovac Biotech on 20 July, involving 9,000 volunteers.
- Mayor of Miami-Dade Carlos A. Giménez announced that restaurants must close their indoor dining areas again due to the rapidly rising coronavirus cases in Florida. This comes as the US death toll reached 130,000.
- US President Donald Trump stated via Twitter that he wants to see all schools in the country reopen after the summer break, despite rising coronavirus cases.
- In Paris, the Louver museum reopened to the public with a reduced capacity and strict social distancing rules.
- Flights between Greece and the UK were revealed to be resuming from 15 July.
- Israeli Prime Minister Benjamin Netanyahu announced that bars, gyms, and events venues will be forced to close with immediate effect as a result of a surge in cases in the country. The Bank of Israel also predicted a six per cent contraction of the country's GDP.
- British sandwich company Pret A Manger announced that a total of thirty stores across the country will close due to the economic aftermath of the coronavirus pandemic, with more than 1,000 jobs expected to be lost. It was revealed that the

company had sales 74 percent lower than in the same period last year, with monthly losses of as much as £20 million.

- Joint United Nations Environment Programme (UNEP) and International Livestock Research Institute (ILRI) report warn that the world can expect to see another animal-to-human transmission by diseases and states that there is still time to prevent further zoonotic pandemics.
- At a High-Level Political Forum to discuss post-pandemic recovery, Mr. Mher Margaryan, Vice-president of the UN Economic and Social Council, announced that the future of the United Nations Sustainable Development Goals would "depend on our policy choices today" on the global resolve to act in solidarity.
- The United Nations Secretary-General warned that the pandemic had laid bare vulnerabilities to "new and emerging forms of terrorism," such as cyberattacks, bioterrorism, and the misuse of digital technology.
- Health authorities in Saudi Arabia announced rules for this year's Hajj pilgrimage to attempt to prevent transmission of COVID-19. Restrictions include the mandatory wearing of face masks, a strict social distancing between all pilgrims during prayers, reduced capacity on public transport, measures to prevent pilgrims from touching the Kaaba, restaurants selling pre-packaged food and drink, compulsory coronavirus tests, and only pilgrims living in Saudi Arabia permitted to travel to Mecca.
- Kenyan President Uhuru Kenyatta revealed his government's plan to reopen the Kenyan economy. International flights are scheduled to resume from 1 August, and travel bans in the cities of Nairobi, Mombasa, and

Mandera will be lifted on 7 July. However, the country's curfew was extended for an additional month.

7 July

- The Australian state of Victoria has reported 191 new cases.
- France reported 13 new deaths, taking the total to 29,933. This figure accounts for a downward revision of the number of nursing home fatalities; the number who died in the country's hospitals increased by 34 to 19,457. The number of fatalities in nursing homes was confirmed to be 10,476, a decrease from the figure of 10,497 reported a week earlier.
- Germany reported 397 new cases and 12 new deaths, bringing the totals to 197,341 and 9,036 respectively, according to data from the Robert Koch Institute.
- India reported 22,252 new cases and 467 new deaths, taking the death toll above 20,000 to 20,160.
- Indonesia reported 1,268 new cases and 68 new deaths, bringing the totals to 66,226 and 3,309, respectively. It was also reported that 30,785 people had recovered so far.
- Iran reported 2,637 new cases, taking the total number of positive cases to 245,688. The country also reported a record daily increase of 200 deaths, bringing the total to 11,931.
- Malaysia has reported six new cases, with the number of active cases at 72 and the total number at 8,674. Five have recovered, bringing the total number of recovered to 8,481. The death toll remains at 121.
- New Zealand has reported two new cases and two new recoveries, bringing the number of active cases to 22 and the number of recovered to 1,492. There have been a total

of 1,536 cases (1,186 confirmed and 350 probable). The death toll has been 22.

- Serbia reported 299 new cases and 13 deaths, bringing the totals to 16,168 and 330, respectively. 110 patients were reported to be in intensive care.
- Singapore has reported 157 new cases, bringing the total to 45,140.
- South Africa reported 8,971 cases, taking a total of over 200,000 to 205,721.
- Russia reported 6,368 new cases and 198 new deaths, bringing the total numbers to 694,230 and 10,494, respectively.
- Ukraine has reported 564 new cases and 21 new deaths, bringing the total numbers to 49,607 and 1,283, respectively; a total of 22,139 patients have recovered.
- The United Kingdom reported 581 new cases, taking the country's total to 286,349. A further 155 deaths were also recorded, bringing the official total to 44,391, although the Office for National Statistics puts the number of excess deaths from COVID-19 over 55,000.
- The United States reported that the total number of cases had passed 3 million.
- Figures from the Office for National Statistics indicate only 22% of people testing positive for COVID-19 had symptoms on the day they were tested.
- Downing Street rejects calls for Boris Johnson to issue an apology after comments the previous day that "too many care homes didn't really follow procedures" over COVID-19, but says what he was saying was that not enough was known about the virus in its early stages.

- Circus performers' call on the UK government to include their industry in the art rescue package unveiled the previous day.
- The World Health Organization announced that it would shortly issue a brief on the modes of transmission of the new coronavirus, including the matter of airborne transmission. Mona Juul, President of the Economic and Social Council, addressed the inaugural meeting of the High-level Political Forum on Sustainable Development, noting that the dramatic impacts of the COVID-19 pandemic had revealed: "weaknesses in our systems and societies," warned that "a new dynamic" was needed to address the negative shocks.
- Brazilian President Jair Bolsonaro tested positive for COVID-19.
- Director of the National Institute of Allergy and Infectious Diseases Anthony Fauci urged the public to wear face masks in public as a result of the surging coronavirus cases in the US. This came as United States President Donald Trump formally withdrew the US from the World Health Organization.
- Organisers of the Republican Party's annual convention in Jacksonville announced that all attendees will be required to have a test for coronavirus before entering the convention.
- The Palestinian National Authority extended the coronavirus lockdown in the West Bank for five days due to rising cases.
- In the United Arab Emirates, Dubai reopened borders to international tourists, with mandatory coronavirus tests on arrival for travellers without proof of a negative test result.
- The Armenian Deputy Minister of Sport Artur Martirosyan announced that Armenian athletes will not participate at the

Commonwealth of Independent States Games in Kazan in September due to public health concerns.

- The German state of Saxony revealed that events with more than 1,000 attendees will be permitted to resume from 1 September.
- Italian Minister of Health Roberto Speranza announced that flights between Italy and Bangladesh will be suspended for a week after several passengers tested positive for coronavirus on a flight from Dhaka to Rome on 6 July.
- Portuguese Prime Minister António Costa revealed that the Portuguese Government is discussing the possibility of a travel corridor to the UK with the British Government after Portugal was initially excluded from the UK's list of safe countries.
- Serbian President Aleksandar Vučić imposed a nationwide curfew from 10 to 13 July due to the rise in coronavirus cases in the country, with Vučić stating that most hospitals in Belgrade were close to capacity. Therefore social gatherings will be reduced to five people indoors and outdoors from 8 July.
- Spanish Transport Minister José Luis Ábalos stated that 1.8 billion euros of financial aid will be provided to transport companies in Spain. It was revealed that the state-owned rail company Renfe Operadora will receive 1 billion euros of the sum, with the remaining to be provided to private companies.
- Victorian Premier Daniel Andrews announced that metropolitan Melbourne and Mitchell Shire would re-enter lockdown from 12 am 9 July for 6 weeks in Australia.
- The New Zealand Government has requested that Air New Zealand and Singapore Airlines manage international

bookings to New Zealand over the next three weeks to ensure that quarantine facilities are not overwhelmed. Air New Zealand had confirmed that 5,500 people are confirmed to travel back to New Zealand with the airline over the next three weeks.

8 July

- Argentina reported a daily record of 3,604 new cases, raising the total number of confirmed cases to 275,003. The death toll was confirmed to be at 1,694.
- Australia reported 134 new cases in the state of Victoria.
- France reported 32 new deaths, bringing the total to 29,965.
- Hong Kong reported 24 new cases, 19 of which were confirmed to be locally transmitted. The total number of cases stands at 1,324, with 7 deaths.
- Iran reported 153 new deaths, bringing the total death toll to over 12,000. It was also reported that the total number of cases had reached 248,379 and that 209,463 have recovered.
- Malaysia has reported three new cases, bringing the number of active cases to 70 and the total number to 8,677. Five patients have been discharged, bringing the total number of recovered to 8,486. The death toll remains at 121.
- Mexico reported 6,995 new cases and 782 new deaths, bringing the total numbers to 275,003 and 32,796, respectively.
- New Zealand has reported one new case, bringing the number of active cases to 23 and the total number to 1,537 (1,187 confirmed and 350 probable). The number of recovered remains 1,492, and the death toll is 22. The latest

case is a 32-year-old man who briefly escaped managed isolation in Auckland before being detained by the authorities.

- Oman reported 1,210 new cases, taking the total of over 50,000 to 50,207. 9 new deaths were also reported, raising the death toll to 233.
- The Philippines reported 2,539 new cases; the highest daily increase recorded thus far. A further 5 deaths were also reported, raising the death toll to 1,314.
- Russia reported 6,562 new cases, taking the total number of cases above 700,000 to 700,792. A further 173 deaths were also reported, bringing the total confirmed death toll to 10,667.
- Singapore has reported 158 new cases, bringing the total to 45,298. In addition, a patient who had COVID-19 died from respiratory arrest.
- Ukraine has reported 807 new cases and 23 new deaths, bringing the total numbers to 50,414 and 1,306, respectively; a total of 23,119 patients have recovered.
- The United Kingdom reported 630 new cases and 126 new deaths, taking the country's official totals to 286,979 and 44,517, respectively.
- Chancellor Rishi Sunak unveils a £30bn spending package aimed at mitigating the economic impact of the COVID-19 pandemic, including a temporary reduction in VAT for the hospitality sector, a scheme to pay firms £1,000 for each employee brought back from furlough, a scheme to get young people into employment, and a temporary rise in the stamp duty threshold.

- McDonald's resumes are serving breakfast at most of its sites. The annual McDonald's Monopoly campaign is postponed to 2021 for the first time in 15 years.
- New UN research published by the United Nations Office on Drugs and Crime warned of a surge in the trafficking of substandard and faulty medical products due to COVID-19.
- Independent UN human rights expert Saad Alfarargi, Special Rapporteur on the Right to Development, at the second day of the High-Level Political Forum on Sustainable Development, stated that the COVID-19 pandemic had resulted in "a serious setback" for the 2030 Agenda for Sustainable Development, urging the prioritisation of the most vulnerable.
- The UN Secretary-General stated at The Global Summit, part of a five-day virtual event organized by the International Labour Organization that decent jobs must fuel the COVID-19 recovery in order to "build back better."
- The Austrian Government-issued travel warnings for the Eastern European countries of Bulgaria, Romania, and Moldova due to the rising numbers of cases there, as well as imported cases being recorded in Austria from those countries. Under the new guidance, all arriving travellers from the listed countries will be required to show documentation of a negative COVID-19 test result or undergo a 14-day quarantine.
- The German pharmaceutical company Merck revealed that it had reached an agreement with the European Union to supply the company's potential COVID-19 vaccine upon request to member states of the EU.

- President of the Government of Catalonia Quim Torra announced that it will be mandatory to wear a face mask anywhere in Catalonia from 10 July, with fines of up to 100 euros if caught without a mask.
- The British Royal Collection Trust announced that some of the residences of Queen Elizabeth II will reopen from 23 July with strict social distancing and hygiene measures in place, as well as the requirement to prebook tickets. The residences named as reopening were Windsor Castle, the Royal Mews and Queen's Gallery of Buckingham Palace, and Holyrood Palace.
- British Chancellor of the Exchequer Rishi Sunak unveiled the British government's plans to mitigate the economic consequences of the coronavirus pandemic. It was announced that a VAT cut would be provided for the hospitality industry, a stamp duty holiday, and an 'eat out to help out' discount on a selected number of restaurants, whereby diners can receive fifty percent off of their meal up to £10 per person from Monday-Wednesday. Sunak also announced that £2 billion will be spent helping 16-25 year-olds find employment, with businesses scheduled to receive £1,000 for each employee brought off of the furlough scheme. The Treasury also revealed a £3 billion green recovery plan to create jobs and encourage businesses to become more environmentally friendly.
- Murtala Muhammed International Airport and Nnamdi Azikiwe International Airport in the Nigerian cities of Lagos and Abuja reopened for domestic flights, with all of the country's airports scheduled to be operational again by 15 July.

- Certain businesses were allowed to reopen in the Sudanese capital of Khartoum, including restaurants, markets, and non-essential shops. However, the nationwide curfew will remain in place for the foreseeable future.
- Brazilian President Jair Bolsonaro vetoed a law requiring the federal government of Brazil to provide indigenous communities with COVID-19, including provisions of drinking water and medication. In response to Bolsonaro testing positive for COVID-19 on 7 July, RecordTV and Empresa Brasil de Comunicação announced that journalists who had interviewed the president would be required to produce evidence of a negative test result before being allowed to resume work.
- Health authorities in Chile announced that some coronavirus lockdown restrictions can be lifted in Los Ríos Region and Aysén Region from 13 July. Under the eased restrictions, non-essential businesses, including theatres and restaurants, will be permitted to reopen at a reduced capacity, and sporting events can resume with a maximum crowd size of fifty people outdoors.
- Governor of New Jersey Phil Murphy announced that wearing face masks in public spaces outdoors will be made mandatory.
- New York City Mayor Bill de Blasio stated that students will not reopen fully after the summer break due to health concerns. Students will only attend physical lessons for at most three days a week, with the remainder of education taking place virtually.

9 July

- Bolivian President Jeanine Áñez tested positive.
- China reported 9 new cases, all of which were imported, raising the total number of cases to 84,910. No further deaths were reported, leaving the death toll at 4,641. 74 people remain hospitalised.
- Germany reported 442 new cases and 12 new deaths, bringing the total numbers to 197,783 and 9,048 respectively, according to data from the Robert Koch Institute.
- Hong Kong reported 42 new cases, 34 of which were confirmed to be domestically transmitted, raising the total number of cases thus far to 1,366. No further deaths were reported, leaving the death toll at 7.
- India reported a daily record of 24,879 newly confirmed cases, raising the total to 767,296 cases. A further 487 deaths were also recorded, bringing the total death toll to 21,129.
- Indonesia reported 2,657 new cases and 58 new deaths, bringing the totals to 70,736 and 3,417, respectively.
- Japan reported 224 new cases in the capital Tokyo, the largest daily increase so far.
- Malaysia has reported six new cases, bringing the total number to 8,683. 13 cases have been discharged, bringing the total number of recovered to 8,499. There are 63 active cases, with two in intensive care and one on ventilator support. The death toll remains at 121.
- Mexico reported 7,280 new cases, the highest daily total so far, and 730 new deaths, bringing the total numbers to 282,283 and 33,526, respectively.

- New Zealand has reported three new cases, bringing the number of active cases to 24 and the total number to 1,540 (1,190 confirmed 350 probable). There were two reported new recoveries, bringing the total number of recovered to 1,494. The death toll remains at 22.
- Nigeria reported 460 new cases, taking the country's total above 30,000 to 30,249. The total death toll was reported to be 684.
- Qatar reported 557 new cases and 4 new deaths, bringing the totals to 102,110 and 142, respectively.
- Singapore has reported 125 new cases, bringing the total to 45,422. In addition, a patient who had COVID-19 died from respiratory arrest.
- Slovakia reported 53 new cases, the biggest increase since April, raising the total to 1,851. It was also reported that the death toll stands at 28, with 1,477 recoveries. The number of active cases was confirmed to be 346, the highest since May 12.
- South Africa reported 13,674 new cases, the highest daily total so far, raising the total number of confirmed cases so far to 238,339. A further 129 deaths were recorded, bringing the total death toll to 3,720; 113,061 patients have recovered. The health department also announced that over two million tests had now been performed.
- South Korea reported 50 new cases, raising the total to 13,293. The death toll remained at 287.
- Ukraine has reported 810 new cases and 21 new deaths, bringing the total numbers to 51,224 and 1,327, respectively; a total of 23,784 patients have recovered.

- The United Kingdom reported 85 new deaths, bringing the total death toll to 44,602. No new deaths were reported in Scotland.
- The United States reported 65,551 new cases, the highest daily amount so far, raising the total number of confirmed cases to over 3.1 million. According to data from Johns Hopkins University, 1,000 deaths were recorded in the last 24 hours, raising the country's death toll to 133,195.
- High street retailers Boots and John Lewis announce job losses because of the COVID-19 pandemic, with Boots cutting 4,000 positions and John Lewis closing eight stores with the loss of 1,300 posts.
- Two sets of data are released that show the number of cases of COVID-19 is falling in England; Office for National Statistics figures estimate one in 3,900 people have the virus, down from one in 2,200 the previous week, while Public Health England figures indicate that cases fell by 25% in the week to 5 July.
- The Institute of Fiscal Studies warns that taxes will have to rise to pay off the support measures put in place by the government.
- Northern Ireland lifts quarantine regulations on arrivals from 50 countries, including France, Italy, Germany, and Spain, effective from 10 July.
- The BBC confirms it will go ahead with plans to end free TV licenses for over-75s from 1 August, except for those on pension credit, a measure it postponed because of the COVID-19 pandemic.
- Pakistani Federal Minister for Education and Professional Training Shafqat Mahmood announced that all schools,

colleges, and universities will reopen on 15 September with strict hygiene measures in place.

- The United Nations Secretary-General called on UN Member States to urgently address the 'unprecedented' impact of coronavirus on Latin America and the Caribbean, as it now had the highest rates of transmission, exacerbating the severe poverty, hunger, unemployment, and inequality in the region.
- The World Food Programme and the UNHCR, the UN refugee agency, issued a joint alert calling attention to even greater food insecurity in Africa because of "aid disruption and rising food prices linked to the COVID-19 crisis".
- Mohammed Ibn Chambas, Special Representative of the Secretary-General and Head of the United Nations Office for West Africa and the Sahel, warned that COVID-19 and climate change were fueling inter-communal violence and terrorist attacks and inflaming tensions in West Africa.
- The World Health Organization announced that an independent inquiry will be launched into the organisation's handling of the coronavirus pandemic following strong criticism and eventual withdrawal from the United States. Director-General Tedros Adhanom that former Prime Minister of New Zealand Helen Clark, and former President of Liberia Ellen Johnson Sirleaf would chair the panel.
- Italian Minister of Health Roberto Speranza announced that Italian borders will be closed to travellers from a list of countries deemed to have unsafe levels of coronavirus transmission. The countries listed were Armenia, Bahrain, Bangladesh, Bosnia & Herzegovina, Brazil, Chile, Dominican Republic, Kuwait, Moldova, North Macedonia, Oman, Panama, and Peru.

- Serbian Prime Minister Ana Brnabić announced that a previously planned weekend curfew would not be enforced as a result of anti-lockdown protests in the capital city of Belgrade; instead, indoor gatherings will be limited to ten individuals, and working hours at restaurants will be reduced.
- President of the Balearic Islands Francina Armengol confirmed that it will be mandatory to wear a face-covering in all public spaces from 13 July, with the only exemptions being for children under six, with fines of up to 100 euros if caught without a mask.
- British Secretary of State for Digital, Culture, Media, and Sports Oliver Dowden announced that certain leisure and beauty businesses will be permitted to reopen later in the month. Outdoor swimming pools will be permitted to reopen on 11 July, with indoor sports facilities and gyms reopening later on 25 July. It was also confirmed that beauty businesses, including tattoo parlours, spas, and tanning salons, can largely reopen from 13 July. However, face treatments will be excluded due to a higher risk of transmission.
- Emirates, the national airline of the United Arab Emirates, announced a further loss of thousands of jobs, including pilots and cabin crew, due to the economic consequences of the coronavirus pandemic.
- The Australian state of Queensland closed its borders to people arriving from Victoria as the city of Melbourne began a new lockdown in response to rising coronavirus cases, with residents given stay-at-home notices for six weeks.

- The Chinese Ministry of Science and Technology announced that it would seek international cooperation to develop vaccines and drugs to treat COVID-19. Chinese authorities also stated that no international sports events will take place for the remainder of the year, with the exception of trials for the 2022 Winter Olympics, to prevent possible imported cases.
- Bolivian President Jeanine Áñez tested positive for COVID-19 and announced that she would continue to work whilst self-isolating at home.
- Mayor of the Brazilian city of Rio de Janeiro, Marcelo Crivella, announced that the city's beaches will only officially reopen when a vaccine for COVID-19 is found.
- The United States Department of Labor revealed that a further 1.3 million Americans applied for unemployment benefits in the last week.
- American coffee company Starbucks announced that face coverings will be mandatory at all stores in the US from 15 July.

10 July

- The World Health Organization reported a record increase in global coronavirus cases, with the total rising by 228,102 in 24 hours.
- The Czech Republic reported 82 new cases, taking the total of over 13,000.
- France reported over 600 new cases for the third consecutive day. 25 new deaths were recorded, taking the total death toll over 30,000 to 30,004.

- Hong Kong reported 38 new cases, raising the total confirmed so far to 1,404. The death toll remains at 7.
- India reported 26,506 new cases, the highest daily number so far.
- Indonesia reported 1,611 new cases and 52 new deaths, bringing the numbers to 72,347 and 3,469, respectively. It was also confirmed that 33,529 patients have recovered.
- Lebanon reported 71 new cases, the highest daily number so far.
- Malaysia has reported 13 new cases, bringing the total number of cases to 8,696. 12 patients have been discharged, bringing the total number of recovered to 8,511. There are 64 active cases, while the death toll remains at 121.
- Namibia reported 52 new cases and its first death, a 45-year-old man. The total number of cases has reached 667.
- New Zealand has reported two new cases, bringing the number of active cases to 23 and the total number to 1,542 (1,192 confirmed and 350 probable). Three new cases were reported, bringing the total number of recovered to 1,497. The death toll remains at 22.
- Serbia reported 386 new cases and 18 new deaths, bringing the total numbers to 386 and 18, respectively.
- Russia reported 6,635 new cases and 174 new deaths, bringing the total numbers to 713,936 and 11,017 respectively, with 489,068 patients having recovered.
- Singapore has reported 191 new cases, bringing the total to 45,613.

- Ukraine has reported 819 new cases and 18 new deaths, bringing the total numbers to 52,043 and 1,345, respectively; a total of 24,800 patients have recovered.
- The United Kingdom reported 48 new deaths, taking the official total to 44,650. No new deaths were recorded in Scotland, Wales, or Northern Ireland.
- The United States reported 69,000 new cases, another daily record, raising the total to 3.18 million, with more than 134,000 deaths confirmed so far.
- Quarantine rules are relaxed for people arriving in the UK from 75 countries and overseas territories.
- Figures released by the National Police Chiefs' Council show that no fines were issued in England and Wales for breach of quarantine rules during the first two weeks after their introduction, while ten people were fined for not wearing face coverings on public transport in the two weeks preceding 22 June.
- As the wearing of face coverings becomes mandatory in shops in Scotland, the UK Government is considering whether to introduce the same rule for shops in England. At the same time, Prime Minister Boris Johnson is seen in public wearing one.
- Bosses at the Birmingham Repertory Theatre, one of the UK's leading production theatres, warn the theatre is at risk of losing 47 of its staff members (about 40% of its workforce) and is in danger of closing because of the economic impact of the COVID-19 pandemic.
- Indian Prime Minister Narendra Modi announced that a nine-day curfew will be imposed in Aurangabad due to a spike in

coronavirus cases. The state of Uttar Pradesh also entered lockdown for two days due to surging cases.

- Malaysian Senior Minister Ismail Sabri Yaakob announced that family entertainment centres, including game arcades, karaoke centres, indoor funfairs, edutainment centres for children, and kids' gymnasiums, will be allowed to resume operations from 15 July.
- The World Health Organization announced that COVID-19 cases globally had more than doubled in the previous six weeks, reaching 12 million.
- United Nations High Commissioner for Human Rights Michelle Bachelet warned that Lebanon was "fast spiralling out of control," resulting in destitution and starvation, due to socioeconomic shocks from the pandemic.
- Vladimir Voronkov, head of the United Nations Office of Counter-Terrorism, echoed the United Nations Secretary-General in stating the "need to keep up the momentum" in terms of multilateral action to counter the global threat of terrorism during the pandemic, which was magnifying the threats.
- European Council President Charles Michel revealed the European Union's plans to aid economic recovery from the coronavirus pandemic. He proposed a 750 billion euro recovery fund, although did not state whether the fund would take the form of grants or loans. However, Finnish Prime Minister Sanna Marin and Swedish Minister for EU Affairs Hans Dahlgren expressed concerns over the potential fund.
- President of Kazakhstan Kassym-Jomart Tokayev warned that the cabinet may be sacked if the coronavirus situation

does not improve in the country by the end of the second nationwide lockdown, imposed on 5 July.

- The Norwegian Government announced that some travel restrictions will be lifted from 15 July, with travel permitted to resume to most countries in the Schengen area (although only some provinces of Sweden are included) and the UK; it was confirmed that the list of safe countries will be reviewed every two weeks.
- Deputy Prime Minister of Russia Tatyana Golikova stated that Russia could begin lifting restrictions on international air travel from 15 July, two weeks earlier than the scheduled date of 1 August. Flights will only be permitted to countries where cases do not exceed 40 per 100,000 people, where the rate of transmission is less than one, and where the average daily increase in cases over the last 14 days is lower than one percent.
- New quarantine measures came into place in England, allowing travellers arriving from a list of 75 countries and all British overseas territories deemed to have a low risk of coronavirus transmission to enter without having to undergo an otherwise mandatory 14-day quarantine in an attempt to boost income for the struggling aviation and hospitality sectors, although the government advised citizens against cruise holidays. Similar measures were implemented in Northern Ireland, with an almost identical list of safe countries. British Prime Minister Boris Johnson also announced that tighter restrictions on the use of face masks might be needed after they were made mandatory in shops in Scotland.

- From today, Northern Ireland allowed businesses, including gyms, playgrounds, cinemas, and arcades, to reopen with strict social distancing and hygiene measures in place. Authorities also introduced legislation requiring people to wear face masks on public transport, with the only exemptions being for people with medical conditions, children under thirteen, and on school transport.
- Australian Prime Minister Scott Morrison stated that the number of Australian citizens allowed to return to the country every day will be halved from 8,000 to 4,000 on 13 July in response to rising cases, most notable in the state of Victoria.
- The Education Bureau of Hong Kong announced that schools will be immediately suspended from 13 July as a result of a spike in domestically transmitted coronavirus cases in the territory.
- Scientific researchers at Japan's Fujita Health University published the results of a potential favipiravir drug developed by Fujifilm to treat COVID-19; results of the tests yielded inconclusive results as to the efficacy of the drug.
- The New Zealand Government has announced that overseas-based victims of the Christchurch mosque shootings would receive special border passes and financial help in order to fly to New Zealand for the duration of the gunman Brenton Tarrant's sentencing, which begins on 24 August.
- The General Statistics Office of Vietnam revealed that the coronavirus pandemic has resulted in 900,000 job losses in the country, with 18 million people receiving a lower income than before the pandemic. Unemployment in Vietnam's

urban communities reportedly rose to the highest level in ten years as a direct result of lockdown restrictions.

- Mayor of Bogotá Claudia López Hernández will raise the Colombian capital's COVID-19 alert level to amber on 13 July, with intensive care units on red alert, due to surging coronavirus cases. López also stated that a "strict quarantine" will be imposed.
- Governor of California Gavin Newsom announced that up to 8,000 prisoners will be released from the state's prisons in an effort to slow the spread of the coronavirus throughout the facilities.
- Players and owners of the National Hockey League in the US and Canada approved an agreement to resume the season from 1 August in Toronto and Edmonton. However, all games will be played without audiences due to the risk of transmission of COVID-19.
- Algerian authorities announced that some travel restrictions will be reimposed to slow the spread of coronavirus. Under the new restrictions, travel will be suspended to and from 29 provinces, including the capital Algiers, for a week. Testing capacity will be increased by allowing all private laboratories to conduct tests.
- Kuwait's Ministry of Health advised the country's citizens against foreign travel due to uncertainties surrounding the coronavirus pandemic and the increased spread of the virus in spite of the various measures implemented by foreign governments.
- Mayor of Bogotá Claudia López Hernández will raise the Colombian capital's COVID-19 alert level to amber on 13 July, with intensive care units on red alert, due to surging

coronavirus cases. López also stated that a "strict quarantine" will be imposed.

- Governor of California Gavin Newsom announced that up to 8,000 prisoners will be released from the state's prisons in an effort to slow the spread of the coronavirus throughout the facilities.
- Players and owners of the National Hockey League in the US and Canada approved an agreement to resume the season from 1 August in Toronto and Edmonton. However, all games will be played without audiences due to the risk of transmission of COVID-19.

11 July

- Australia reported 216 new cases in the state of Victoria.
- Brazil reported 45,000 new cases, taking the total to 1.8 million. 1,200 new deaths were also recorded, taking the death toll over 70,000 to 70,400.
- India reported a new high (for the third consecutive day) of 27,114 daily confirmed cases, taking a total of over 800,000 to 820,916. 519 new deaths were also reported, raising that total to 22,123.
- Italy reported 188 new cases, a third of which were in the region of Lombardy, bringing the total to 242,827. 7 new deaths were also reported, raising the total to 34,945. The total number of active cases fell to 13,303; over 5.95 million tests have been performed.
- Lebanon reported a daily record of 86 new cases, raising the country's total death toll to 2,168. A total of 36 deaths have been reported.

- Malaysia has reported eight new cases (four imported cases), bringing the total number to 8,704. There are 67 active cases, with three in intensive care and two on ventilator support. Four patients have recovered, bringing the total number of recovered to 8,515. The country also reported one new death, bringing the total to 122.
- Mexico reported 6,094 new cases and 539 new deaths, bringing the total numbers to 295,268 and 34,730, respectively.
- New Zealand has reported one new case, bringing the number of active cases to 24 and the total number to 1,543 (1,193 confirmed and 350 probable). The number of recovered remains at 1,497, while the death toll remains at 24.
- Palestine recorded 436 new cases, bringing the total number confirmed thus far to 5,827. A further 5 deaths were recorded, raising the total death toll to 35. 829 people have recovered.
- The Philippines reported 1,387 new cases, raising the total to 54,222. 12 new deaths were also recorded.
- Russia reported 6,611 new cases and 188 new deaths, bringing the total numbers so far to 720,547 and 11,205, respectively.
- Singapore has reported 170 new cases, bringing the total to 45,783.
- South Africa reported 13,497 new cases and 3,971 new deaths, bringing the total numbers to 264,184 and 3,971, respectively.
- Turkey reported 1,016 new cases and 21 new deaths, bringing the total numbers to 211,981 and 5,344,

respectively. It was also announced that 1,334 patients have recovered, bringing the total number of recoveries to 193,217.

- Ukraine has reported 800 new cases and 27 new deaths, bringing the total numbers to 52,843 and 1,372, respectively; a total of 25,661 patients have recovered.
- The United Kingdom reported 820 new cases and 148 new deaths, taking the official totals to 288,953 and 44,798, respectively. It was also announced that 153,667 tests had been performed in the last 24 hours.
- The United States reported 66,528 new cases and 760 new deaths, raising the totals to 3,242,073 and 134,729, respectively, according to data from Johns Hopkins University. Florida reported the largest daily increase in cases in a single state so far, with 15,299 positive cases confirmed.
- Parts of The Health Protection (Coronavirus, Restrictions) (No. 2) (England) (Amendment) Regulations 2020 come into effect, allowing outdoor swimming pools and water parks to re-open. Operators of outdoor swimming pools, many of the community groups and charities, criticise the UK government's timing, citing a lack of preparation time that has made a short summer season "unviable."
- Belgium includes Leicester on its "red zone" list, meaning anyone who has recently visited the city will be required to quarantine for 14 days on arrival in Belgium.
- As part of World Population Day, the United Nations Secretary-General highlighted that the pandemic had deepened "existing inequalities and vulnerabilities, particularly for women and girls,"." At the same time, the

United Nations Population Fund warned of seven million unintended pregnancies and approximately 31 million additional cases of gender-based violence to come.

- The United Nations warned that in Myanmar, the COVID-19 lockdown had laid bare the "stigmatization, discrimination and harassment faced by many LGBTQI people, particularly in rural areas," and committed to assisting the community.
- Authorities in the Indian-administered territory of Jammu and Kashmir are reportedly considering imposing a regional lockdown after the number of confirmed coronavirus cases there passed 10,000.
- India's Drug Controller General granted approval for the drug tocilizumab developed by Indian biopharmaceutical company Biocon Ltd to be used in emergency situations on moderately to severely affected coronavirus patients.
- Magic Kingdom and Animal Kingdom at Walt Disney World Resort in Orlando, Florida reopened to the public with a reduced capacity, mandatory temperature checks on arrival, hand sanitising stations throughout the park, and the requirement to wear a face mask. It had been previously announced that all live performances would be suspended when the park reopens to lower the risk of transmission.
- United States Ambassador to the United Nations Andrew Bromberg stated that the US Government welcomed the inquiry launched by the World Health Organization into the origins of the coronavirus pandemic in China.
- The Treefort Music Fest in Boise, Idaho, which initially had been postponed to September 2020, was further postponed to September 2021 and March 2022.

- The Bulgarian Football Union announced that the start of the First Professional Football League's season will be postponed by two weeks due to public health concerns relating to coronavirus, with a new start date of 7 August.
- Researchers at the Germany's University of Tübingen announced that 4,000 volunteers have registered to take part in clinical trials for a potential COVID-19 vaccine, which began in June.
- Swiss football club FC Zürich announced that the team's next two games had been cancelled after they were placed into quarantine until 17 July due to multiple cases of COVID-19 being reported amongst the team's players and staff including defender Mirlind Kryeziu.
- President of Iran Hassan Rouhani stated that all weddings should be cancelled due to the risk of coronavirus transmission, prompting authorities in the capital city of Tehran to close all wedding and funeral venues. Rouhani also stated that Iran could not close its economy again, largely as a result of international sanctions.
- Crown Prince of Dubai Hamdan bin Mohammed Al Maktoum announced a 1.5 billion dirham economic stimulus package to aid Dubai's financial recovery from the coronavirus pandemic.
- A report revealed that the national airline of the United Arab Emirates, Emirates, has reduced its workforce by 10 percent during the COVID-19 pandemic, with the loss of over 9,000 jobs, after the company temporarily suspended all operations due to public health concerns.

12 July

- The World Health Organisation reported a new record of 230,370 positive cases confirmed in a single day worldwide.
- Argentina reported 2,657 new cases, taking the total number of confirmed cases above 100,000 to 100,166. The country's death toll stands at 1,845.
- Australia reported 273 new cases and 1 new death in the state of Victoria.
- Brazil reported 631 new deaths, raising the country's total number of deaths to 72,100. The number of confirmed cases rose to 1,864,681.
- China reported 7 new cases, none of which were domestically transmitted, raising the total number of confirmed cases to 83,594. No further deaths were reported, leaving the total death toll at 4,634.
- Germany reported 282 new cases and 3 new deaths, raising the total numbers to 198,804 and 9,063, respectively.
- Greece reported 41 new cases, raising the country's total to 3,772. No new deaths were reported; the death toll stands at 193.
- India reported 28,637 new cases, the highest daily total so far, raising the number of infections to 849,553. A further 551 deaths were also reported, raising the total to 22,674.
- Lebanon reported a record of 166 new cases, raising the total so far to over 2,000.
- Malaysia has reported 14 new cases (three imported and 11 community transmissions), bringing the total number of cases to 8,718. There have been four recoveries while the death toll remains at 122.

- Mexico reported 4,482 new cases and 276 new deaths, bringing the total numbers to 299,750 and 35,006, respectively.
- New Zealand has reported one new case, bringing the number of active cases to 25 and the total number to 1,544 (1,194 confirmed and 350 probable). The number of recovered remains at 1,497, while the death toll remains at 24.
- Russia reported 6,615 new cases and 130 new deaths, bringing the total numbers to 727,162 and 11,335, respectively.
- Singapore has reported 178 new cases, bringing the total to 45,961.
- South Korea reported 44 new cases, 21 of which were domestically transmitted, raising the confirmed number of cases to 13,417. 1 new death was also recorded, raising the total death toll to 289.
- Syria reported 4 new cases in Idlib Governorate.
- Ukraine has reported 678 new cases and 11 new deaths, bringing the total numbers to 53,521 and 1,383, respectively; a total of 26,118 patients have recovered.
- The United Kingdom reported 650 new cases and 21 new deaths, raising the total numbers to 289,603 and 44,819, respectively. No new deaths were reported in Scotland or Wales.
- The United States reported a new daily record of 66,528 cases and 760 new deaths, raising the totals to 3,242,073 and 134,729, respectively, according to data from Johns Hopkins University.

- High Street fashion retailer Primark says it will not take advantage of the Jobs Retention Bonus announced by Chancellor Rishi Sunak. The company placed 30,000 of its employees on furlough during the pandemic but has since brought them all back to work and would have been entitled to £30m under the scheme.
- As part of its response to the pandemic, the International Monetary Fund called for tax systems to be reformed, including to reduce tax avoidance and tax evasion reduced to ensure an equitable economic recovery.
- Governor of Okinawa Prefecture Denny Tamaki urged American military officials to take tougher preventative measures and have greater transparency after 61 military personnel tested positive for COVID-19 at two different Marine Corps bases, Air Station Futenma and Camp Hansen, in a matter of days. US military officials responded by placing the bases into quarantine.
- The Taipei Film Festival in Taiwan went ahead despite the coronavirus pandemic, making it the first in-person film festival to be held worldwide in 2020.
- Health authorities in the Brazilian state of Santa Catarina announced that a football match between Associação Chapecoense de Futebol and Avaí FC would be cancelled after 14 players tested positive for COVID-19.
- In the United States, a Major League Soccer game between D.C. United and Toronto FC was postponed after one of the players tested positive for COVID-19.
- South African President Cyril Ramaphosa reinstated a law prohibiting the sale of alcohol to reduce the number of people admitted to hospitals with alcohol-related injuries in

order to increase capacity for treating coronavirus patients over concerns of potential shortages of hospital beds in the country. A night curfew was also reinstated to reduce traffic-related accidents, and masks were made mandatory in public.

- King Abdullah II of Jordan announced that Jordan has brought the coronavirus pandemic under control and can now prioritise the reopening of the country's economy after unemployment rose to over 19 percent in the first quarter of the year.
- The Palestinian National Authority announced that a night-time curfew will be imposed in the West Bank due to rising coronavirus cases. Bethlehem, Hebron, Nablus, and Ramallah have suspended all travel for four days, with travel between provinces strictly prohibited for two weeks.
- The Abu Dhabi Fund for Development in the United Arab Emirates suspended debt service repayments for several countries and companies due to the economic consequences of the coronavirus pandemic.
- Hungarian authorities announced that border restrictions will be tightened from 15 July due to rising coronavirus cases in various parts of the world. Under the new restrictions, countries with higher rates of transmission will be divided into "yellow" and "red" categories, with travellers arriving from "yellow" countries being required to undergo a mandatory 14-day quarantine, with borders closed to travellers from "red" countries; Hungarian citizens returning from "red" countries must enter quarantine and produce two negative test results before being permitted to leave.
- Prime Minister of Israel Benjamin Netanyahu announced that immediate financial aid will be provided to citizens affected

by the coronavirus pandemic, including disbursements of up to 7,500 shekels to the self-employed in response to growing criticism of the Israeli Government's handling of the pandemic.

- Health officials in the Spanish regions of Galicia and the Basque Country introduced strict safety measures to allow voting in the 2020 Galician regional election and 2020 Basque regional election to go ahead. Voters were required to wear face masks and adhere to a strict 1.5 metre social distance.
- In the United Kingdom, 200 employees at a farm in Herefordshire were forced to self-isolate after 73 individuals tested positive for COVID-19.
- Researchers at Chulalongkorn University in Bangkok announced that human trials of a potential vaccine for COVID-19 will begin with 10,000 volunteers in November, with the aim of producing by the end of 2021.

13 July

- China reported 3 new cases, and 5 new asymptomatic cases, raising the total number of confirmed cases to 83,605. The death toll remains at 4,634.
- France reported that the number of hospitalised COVID-19 patients has decreased from 7,062 to 6,983, with the number in intensive care falling from 496 to 492.
- Germany reported 159 new cases and 1 death, raising the total numbers to 198,963 and 9,064, respectively, according to data from the Robert Koch Institute.
- India reported 28,701 new cases and 500 new deaths, raising the total death toll to 23,174.

- Indonesia reported 1,282 new cases and 50 new deaths, bringing the total numbers to 76,981 and 3,656, respectively.
- Malaysia has reported seven new cases, bring the number of active cases to 83 and the total number to 8,725. There has been one recovery, bring the total number of recovered to 8,520 cases. The death toll remains at 122.
- Mexico reported 4,695 new cases and 485 new deaths, raising the total numbers to 304,435 and 35,491, respectively.
- New Zealand has reported no new cases. The number of active cases remains 25, with the total number remaining at 1,544 (1,194 confirmed and 350 probable). The number of recovered remains at 1,497, while the death toll remains at 22.
- The Philippines reported 2,124 new cases and a new daily high of 162 deaths, raising the total numbers to 56,259 and 1,534, respectively.
- Singapore has reported 322 new cases, bringing the total to 46,282.
- South Korea reported 62 new cases, 19 of which were domestically transmitted, raising the total number confirmed so far to 13,479. No further deaths were reported, leaving the death toll at 289.
- Ukraine has reported 602 new cases and 15 new deaths, bringing the total numbers to 54,133 and 1,398, respectively; a total of 26,503 patients have recovered.

- The United Kingdom reported 11 new deaths, raising the official death toll to 44,830.

- The United States reported 60,469 new cases and 312 new deaths, raising the country's totals to 3,296,599 and 134,884, respectively.
- The remainder of The Health Protection (Coronavirus, Restrictions) (No. 2) (England) (Amendment) Regulations 2020 comes into effect, allowing the re-opening of nail bars and salons, tanning booths and salons, spas and beauty salons, massage parlours, tattoo parlours, and body and skin piercing services.
- The Government of Sri Lanka ordered all state schools in the country to close due to a rise in coronavirus cases, with private schools strongly encouraged to close as well.
- Irish Minister for Tourism, Culture, Arts, Gaeltacht, Sport, and Media Catherine Martin stated that authorities were considering introducing tighter measures on arriving international travellers after criticism from opposition politicians, including the possibility of making it mandatory to undergo a 14-day quarantine, which is currently only recommended.
- President of Kazakhstan Kassym-Jomart Tokayev announced that the country's coronavirus lockdown will be extended by a further two weeks until the end of July and that struggling families will be able to access financial aid from the government.
- A local court in the Spanish Province of Lleida in Catalonia suspended the stay-at-home order imposed on the province by health officials despite rising coronavirus cases.
- British Prime Minister Boris Johnson announced that face coverings will be compulsory in all shops and supermarkets in England from 24 July, with fines of up to £100 for those

who do not comply with the new rules. However, children under 11 and those with certain medical conditions will be exempt.

- In Canada, Premier of Ontario Doug Ford announced that the province will enter the third stage of reopening from 17 July, with nearly all businesses and public spaces being permitted to reopen, as well as allowing gatherings of up to fifty people indoors and a hundred people outdoors, although a strict social distance of at least two metres must be maintained.
- Authorities in Honduras extended the country's curfew by a week in an attempt to control the spread of coronavirus.
- Governor of California Gavin Newsom announced that all restaurants, museums, leisure centres, bars, and cinemas must close across the state due to surging coronavirus cases, with places of worship, gyms, shopping centres, and salons being forced to close in the worst-affected counties. In response, the Los Angeles Unified School District and San Diego Unified School District announced that all education will resume online after the summer break in August.
- Organisers of the 2020 Chicago Marathon, scheduled to be held on 11 October, cancelled the event in response to rising coronavirus cases in the US. Scheduled participants offered the choice of either receiving a refund or deferring their place to a future event.
- The Walt Disney Company announced that Hong Kong Disneyland will be temporarily closed again from 15 July due to rising coronavirus cases in the city. However, all on-site hotels will remain open with limited services available.

- Organisers of the 2020 Hong Kong Book Fair postponed the event, scheduled to be held from 15 July, after the Hong Kong Government announced that large public gatherings will be banned due to rising coronavirus cases in the city.
- The United Nations launched its annual State of Food Security and Nutrition in the World report, which estimates that "130 million more people may face chronic hunger by the end of this year", with the United Nations Secretary-General noting that In much of the world, "hunger remains deeply entrenched and is rising." With United Nations estimates of 1 billion children being outside schooling due to the pandemic, Audrey Azoulay, Director-General of UNESCO, highlighted the need to ensure education for refugee children.
- South African health officials announced that a curfew will be reimposed from 20 July and that face masks will be mandatory in all indoor spaces and vehicles in an attempt to slow the spread of coronavirus in the country.
- The International Monetary Fund warned that the Middle East and North Africa region could face a steeper recession than previously predicted as a result of the pandemic.
- Tunisian Investment Minister Slim Azzabi revealed that the country's economy is predicted to contract by 6.5 percent in 2020 as a direct result of the coronavirus pandemic.

14 July

- Algeria reported 527 new cases; the highest daily increase reported so far, 10 new deaths, and 337 new recoveries.
- Chile reported 1,836 new cases, the lowest daily increase in 63 days, raising the total number of infections to 319,493. The death toll rose to 7,069.
- China reported 6 new cases, all imported, raising the total number of cases to 83,611. No further deaths were reported, leaving the death toll at 4,634.
- Germany reported 412 new cases and 4 new deaths, bringing the total numbers to 199,375 and 9,068, respectively.
- Hong Kong reported 48 new cases, 40 of which were domestically transmitted, raising the total number of confirmed cases to over 1,500. The death toll remains at 8.
- India reported 28,498 new cases and 553 new deaths, bringing the total numbers to 906,752 and 23,727, respectively.
- Iran reported 179 new deaths, raising the total number of fatalities to 13,211. 2,521 new cases were also recorded, raising the total number to 262,173.
- Israel reported 1,681 new cases, the highest daily increase reported so far. 3 new deaths were reported, raising the death toll to 368. There are currently 177 patients in a serious condition, with 55 on ventilators, with a total of 21,118 active cases.
- Malaysia has reported four new cases, bringing the total number of cases to 8,729. There are currently 83 cases, with four in intensive care and two on ventilator support. Four

have recovered, bringing the total number of recovered to 8,524. The death toll remains at 122.

- New Zealand has reported one new case, bringing the number of active cases to 25 and the total number to 1,545 (1,195 confirmed and 350 probable). There was one new recovery, bringing the total to 1,498. The death toll remains at 22.
- The Philippines reported 634 new cases and 6 new deaths, bringing the total numbers to 57,545 and 1,603, respectively.
- Russia reported 6,428 new cases and 175 new deaths, bringing the total numbers to 739,947 and 11,614, respectively.
- Singapore has reported 347 new cases, bringing the total to 46,629. Another death was later confirmed, bringing the total to 27.
- Spain reported 666 new cases from around 120 different outbreaks, raising the total confirmed so far to 256,619.
- Ukraine has reported 638 new cases and 14 new deaths, bringing the total numbers to 54,771 and 1,412, respectively; a total of 27,154 patients have recovered.
- The United Kingdom reported 398 new lab-confirmed cases and 138 new deaths, bringing the official totals to 291,373 and 44,968, respectively. No further deaths were reported in Scotland.
- A report commissioned by the UK's chief scientific adviser, Sir Patrick Vallance, produces estimates for potential COVID-19 deaths in a deadly second wave scenario over the coming winter, with best and worst-case outcomes depending on the level of action taken to control the virus. The report forecasts a figure of between 24,500 and 251,000

hospital deaths, with a peak in January and February 2021, but stresses the figures are forecasts and not predictions and do not take factors such as the development of a vaccine into account.

- The UK government announces that the wearing of face coverings will become compulsory in shops and supermarkets in England from 24 July. Those who fail to do so will face a fine of up to £100. Health Secretary Matt Hancock says the move will "give people more confidence to shop safely and enhance protections for those who work in shops."
- Figures from the Office for National Statistics show that UK economic recovery was at 1.8% in May 2020 compared to the previous month, a smaller amount than was expected.
- Director of the United States Centers for Disease Control and Prevention Robert R. Redfield stated that the coronavirus pandemic in the US could be controlled in as little as eight weeks if all Americans wore face masks.
- Secretary-General of the United Nations António Guterres warned that the pandemic has the potential to push the world back "years and even decades" in terms of economic progression, with estimates suggesting 100 million people could be forced into extreme poverty during the pandemic.
- Health authorities in Hong Kong announced a tightening of lockdown restrictions after several days of rising coronavirus cases, raising concerns of a possible second wave of infections. Under the new restrictions, face masks were made mandatory on public transport with fines of up to 5,000 Hong Kong dollars if caught without one; non-essential businesses including gyms and entertainment venues were forced to close, and restaurants were told to close indoor

dining areas. Social gatherings were also reduced to a maximum of four people.

- Health authorities in the Japanese capital of Tokyo revealed that they urgently needed to contact around 800 people who had attended productions at the Theatre Molière after several cases of coronavirus were reported in the cast and audience.
- In the Philippines, Secretary of the Interior and Local Government Eduardo Año announced that the Philippine National Police will conduct house-to-house searches for coronavirus patients to prevent the further spread of the virus in the country.
- Data from Singapore's Ministry of Trade and Industry suggests that the country's economy contracted by a record of 41 percent in the second financial quarter between April and June, as a direct result of the coronavirus pandemic, meaning that the country's economy entered its first recession since the 2008 financial crisis.
- Authorities in Oman announced that citizens will soon travel abroad, although no date was specified. International travel will require citizens to register with authorities and undergo a mandatory quarantine on return; it was also revealed that the lockdowns in Dhofar Governorate and on Masirah Island will be maintained due to high numbers of coronavirus cases.
- Authorities in territory controlled by Houthi rebels in Yemen announced an easing of coronavirus lockdown restrictions, allowing the reopening of restaurants, parks, and wedding venues whilst encouraging the public to maintain a social distance and use hand sanitiser regularly.

- French President Emmanuel Macron announced that face masks will be mandatory in all indoor areas from 1 August.
- Head of the German Chancellery and coordinator of the German government's response to the COVID-19 pandemic Helge Braun announced that authorities are considering introducing local travel bans to prevent the second wave of coronavirus infections and that social distancing and the wearing of face masks in public will likely remain in place for the next few months.
- Hungarian Prime Minister Viktor Orbán announced that he will veto the pandemic recovery fund proposed by the European Union if poorer countries receive less funding or conditions such as migration policy conformity are imposed.
- Italian Minister of Health Roberto Speranza revealed that restrictive measures will remain in place until August to avoid a possible second wave of coronavirus infections. The mandatory 14-day quarantine for all travellers arriving in Italy from outside the European Union will be maintained.
- Health authorities in the Spanish autonomous community of Catalonia re-imposed a stay-at-home order in the city of Lleida and several surrounding towns for 15 days after a surge in coronavirus infections. However, it must be improved by a judge to come into effect. Under the new restrictions, residents will only be permitted to leave their homes for essential reasons, and non-essential businesses will be forced to close, with social gatherings of more than ten people also prohibited.
- Organisers of the 2020 Swiss Indoors tennis tournament cancelled the event due to concerns over coronavirus.

- The national rail operator of Turkmenistan, Türkmendemirýollary, announced that all trains will be halted for a week from 16 to 23 July after some media outlets reported that the first coronavirus cases had been identified in the country.
- The South African Democratic Teachers Union urged education authorities to close all schools in South Africa due to the rapidly rising coronavirus cases in the country, with general secretary Mukwena Maluleke highlighting evidence suggesting that cases have been rising quicker since the reopening of schools and that schools remaining open in the current situation put students and staff at a greater risk of contracting COVID-19.
- Human Rights Watch urged the National Bank of Cambodia and the Cambodian Government to suspend debt collection and interest accruals for those who can no longer make the payments as a result of the economic impacts of the coronavirus pandemic, arguing that debt relief measures provided to struggling citizens by micro-loan providers have not been successful.
- The Indian city of Bangalore returned to lockdown for a week as a result of surging coronavirus cases in the country. Under the new restrictions, all non-essential shops were forced to close, with essential shops and pharmacies only permitted to open in the morning. All public transport and travel to different regions was also suspended.
- Malaysian Foreign Minister Hishammuddin Hussein and Singaporean Foreign Minister Vivian Balakrishnan have announced that cross-border travel and traffic between the two countries will resume on 10 August 2020.

- As part of the Ministerial Segment of the High-level Political Forum on Sustainable Development, the United Nations Secretary-General admitted that the planet was not on track year to deliver the Sustainable Development Goals by 2030, stating that "our world is in turmoil" due to the pandemic being "a massive global challenge" and noting that there were 12 million infections, 550,000 deaths, hundreds of millions of jobs lost, and the sharpest decline in per capita income since 1870, with approximately 265 million people facing food insecurity by the end of 2020, double the number before the pandemic. The Secretary-General called on the Member States to "turn the tide."
- In response to a press question, Dr. Michael Ryan, Executive Director of the WHO Health Emergencies Programme, called for the issue of school reopenings to be decided as part of comprehensive, data-driven COVID-19 public health strategies rather than politically-driven decision-making processes.
- United Nations Deputy Secretary-General Amina Mohammed emphasized the importance of the 'Women Rise for All' UN forum in shaping leadership in pandemic response and recovery.
- Qu Dongyu, Director-General of the Food and Agriculture Organization, launched its comprehensive COVID-19 Response and Recovery Programme to ward off a global food emergency during and after the pandemic and to provide "medium to long-term development responses for food security and nutrition," costing an initial $1.2 billion investment.

15 July

- Malaysia has reported five new cases, bringing the number of active cases to 86 and the total number to 8,734. Two people were discharged, bringing the total number of recovered to 8,526. The death toll remains at 122.
- New Zealand has reported two new cases, bringing the number of active cases to 27 and the total number to 1,547 (1,197 confirmed and 350 probable). The number of recovered remains at 1,498, while the death toll remains at 22.
- Singapore has reported 249 new cases, bringing the total to 46,878.
- Ukraine has reported 836 new cases and 15 new deaths, bringing the total numbers to 55,607 and 1,427, respectively; a total of 28,131 patients have recovered.
- Prime Minister Boris Johnson confirms an independent inquiry will be held into the handling of the pandemic but says it would not be right to devote "huge amounts of official time" to an inquiry while the pandemic is ongoing.
- A temporary cut in Value-added tax worth £4bn comes into force until 12 January 2021 as a means of helping the food and hospitality industries. Nando's, Pret a Manger, KFC, and McDonald's are among the firms to announce price reductions as a result.
- Online retailer ASOS says it will repay furlough cash it received from the UK government after sales increased by 10% to £1bn in the four months up to 30 June.
- Indian Prime Minister Narendra Modi revealed that several cities and states, including the cities of Bangalore, Pune, and Shillong and the states of Uttar Pradesh, Tamil Nadu, and

Assam, will have coronavirus lockdowns re-imposed due to surging infections in the country.

- Primary and secondary schools in Malaysia were permitted to reopen in stages due to a sustained drop in coronavirus infections in the country, with strict hygiene measures in place.
- International flights were permitted to resume from airports in Senegal after being suspended for four months. All arriving travellers are required to provide evidence of a negative COVID-19 test result received in the last week; the country's land borders and ports remain closed.
- The United States Department of Health and Human Services announced that the American government will take direct control of all coronavirus-related data from the Centers for Disease Control and Prevention, which has been criticised for its slow and inconsistent reporting throughout the pandemic. All information will be sent to computer databases in Washington, D.C...
- Managers at the American retail corporation Walmart announced that customers will be required to wear face masks in-store from 20 July amid rising coronavirus cases in the US.
- Organisers of the 2021 Rose Parade, scheduled to be held in Pasadena, California, on 1 January, cancelled the event due to concerns over coronavirus; this is the first time the event has been cancelled since World War II.
- The Chinese Ministry of Culture and Tourism announced an easing of restrictions on domestic tourism, with popular destinations allowed to increase visitor capacity from 30

percent to 50 percent, and inter-province tours also permitted to resume.

- Authorities in the Japanese capital of Tokyo raised the city's coronavirus alert level to the highest level following a surge in infections. Governor Yuriko Koike urged residents to avoid non-essential travel outside of Tokyo and also to avoid visiting businesses that have not implemented suitable preventative measures for COVID-19.
- New Zealand Prime Minister Jacinda Ardern released the Government's COVID-19 response framework, which would involve localised lockdowns in the event there was another community-wide outbreak of COVID-19.
- Health officials in the South Korean city of Pyeongtaek have asked the country's government to request pre-arrival coronavirus tests for American soldiers stationed at Camp Humphreys following a spike in infections amongst American military personnel there.
- Organisers of the 2020 Mercuries Taiwan Masters golf tournament cancelled the event, scheduled to be held from 17 to 20 September, due to coronavirus health concerns and international travel restrictions on players and audiences, with the event now scheduled to be played in the same time period in 2021.
- The World Health Organization and UNICEF called for immediate efforts to vaccinate all children in order to avoid the pandemic worsening access, a problem affecting over 100 countries. United Nation Youth Envoy Jayathma Wickramanayake, along with the World Health Organization and the UN Children's Fund, considered via webinar "how young people can maintain good mental health and a sense of wellbeing" during the pandemic.

- Austria's Federal Ministry for European and International Affairs lifted warnings currently advising against non-essential travel to the Italian region of Lombardy after a decline in the number of coronavirus cases.
- The postponed 2020 North Macedonian parliamentary election was held with several coronavirus measures implemented, including strict social distancing rules and the mandatory wearing of face masks.
- Authorities on the Spanish island of Mallorca announced that bars and nightclubs popular with foreign tourists in Magaluf and Las Palmas must close to prevent large gatherings of people behaving in a disorderly manner.
- British Prime Minister Boris Johnson announced that an independent inquiry into the government's handling of the coronavirus pandemic will be held to attempt to prevent a potentially deadlier second wave of the virus. However, Johnson stated that "now is not the time" due to the current situation in the country. Health Secretary Matt Hancock also stated that face coverings will not be compulsory in offices.

16 July

- Australia reported 317 cases, a new daily record, and 2 new deaths in the state of Victoria.
- India reported a daily high of 32,695 new cases, taking the country's total number of confirmed cases to 968,876. A further 1,118 deaths were reported, raising the death toll to 24,915. There are currently 331,146 active cases, and 612,815 patients have recovered.
- Indonesia reported 1,574 new cases and 76 new deaths, bringing the total numbers to 81,668 and 3,873, respectively.

- Malaysia has reported three new cases (one Malaysia and two foreigners), bringing the total number to 8,737. There are 77 active cases, with three in intensive care and one on ventilator support. 12 patients were discharged, bringing the total number of recovered to 8,538. The death toll remains at 122.
- Malta has not reported a new case in a week, with a total of 4 active cases.
- New Zealand has reported one new case, bringing the number of active cases to 27 and the total number to 1,548 (1,198 confirmed and 350 probable). One person also recovered, bringing the total number of recovered to 1,499. The death toll remains at 22.
- Pakistan reported 2,145 new cases, raising the total number confirmed so far to 257,915. A further 153 deaths were also reported, the lowest daily number in over a month, raising the total death toll to 5,426.
- Russia reported 6,428 new cases and 167 new deaths, bringing the total numbers to 752,797 and 11,937, respectively.
- Singapore has reported 248 new cases, bringing the total to 47,126.
- Ukraine has reported 848 new cases and 18 new deaths, bringing the total numbers to 56,455 and 1,445, respectively; a total of 28,931 patients have recovered.
- The United Kingdom reported 642 new cases and 66 new deaths, raising the official numbers to 292,552 and 45, 119. All of the new deaths had underlying medical conditions; Scotland recorded its first death in eight days.

- The United States passed 3.5 million total cases, with more than 137,000 deaths, according to data from Johns Hopkins University.
- The National Cyber Security Centre accuses Russian spies of targeting organisations developing COVID-19 vaccines in the United Kingdom, United States, and Canada in order to steal information relating to their work.
- Figures released by the UK government show the number of workers on UK payrolls fell by 649,000 from March to June. Still, unemployment did not increase as much as feared because many companies took advantage of the Coronavirus Job Retention Scheme.
- Speaking to the House of Commons Scientific Advisory Committee, the UK's Chief Medical Officer Sir Patrick Vallance says there is "absolutely no reason" to change the advice about working from home. It remains a "perfectly good option" for many.
- Health Secretary Matt Hancock announces that the Leicester local lockdown is to be extended. The boundaries are redrawn so that only the Leicester unitary authority plus the borough of Oadby and Wigston are now included in the travel and business restrictions, with the other areas of Leicestershire being released. A review of the situation was set for 1 August.
- Authorities in the Indian-controlled territory of Kashmir announced that Hindus will be allowed to make the pilgrimage to the holy Amarnath Temple in the Himalayas, due to begin on 21 July. However, only 500 pilgrims a day will be permitted to ensure social distancing measures can be enforced.

- Chinese pharmaceutical company Fosun Pharmaceutical received permission from health authorities to begin the first phase of human trials of the company's potential COVID-19 vaccine using technology developed by the German company BioNTech.
- The National Bureau of Statistics of China revealed that the Chinese GDP increased by 3.2 percent in the second fiscal quarter of 2020 despite the coronavirus pandemic, attributed to the lifting of lockdown restrictions and the reopening of factories.
- United States Secretary of Homeland Security Chad Wolf announced that the American borders with Mexico and Canada will remain closed to non-essential travel until at least 20 August to prevent further spread of COVID-19, with Canadian authorities stating that there may be increased surveillance and enforcement along the country's border.
- Governor of Arkansas Asa Hutchinson and Governor of Colorado Jared Polis announced that it will now be mandatory to wear a face mask in public in Arkansas and Colorado. The Governor of Georgia, Brian Kemp, continues to receive criticism for preventing cities in the state from mandating the wearing of face masks in public, arguing that cities do not have the statutory authority to make such a decision.
- Governor of New York Andrew Cuomo stated that New York City is "not ready" to reopen shopping centres and museums even if authorities move into the next phase of reopening. Cuomo stated that no additional indoor activity will open in the state during the fourth phase of reopening due to the risk of coronavirus transmission.

- The US Centers for Disease Control and Prevention extended the ban on cruise ships sailing in U.S. waters to 30 September due to the rapidly rising coronavirus cases in the country.
- President of Venezuela Nicolás Maduro announced that coronavirus restrictions will be tightened in the cities of Caracas and Cumaná, and the states of Miranda and Zulia following a rise in infections. Under the "Level 1 - Radical Quarantine" measures, people can only leave their homes for essential reasons, and all non-essential businesses were forced to close.
- Mark Lowcock, the United Nations' most senior humanitarian official, warned that the COVID-19 pandemic and resulting recession were set to cause the first increase in global poverty in three decades, pushing 265 million people to the point of starvation by the end of 2020, with an appeal to the G20 for $10.3 billion to fight the pandemic in 63 low-income countries.
- The United Nations Human Right Council noted that there was a global rise in women prisoners that was accelerating faster than the rate of male prisoners and that COVID measures were "making sentences worse."
- The European Union removed Montenegro and Serbia from the list of countries deemed safe to allow non-essential travel to as a result of rising coronavirus infections in the two countries, effectively re-introducing a travel ban.
- Hungarian Minister of the Prime Minister's Office Gergely Gulyás announced that celebrations scheduled for Hungary's national day on 20 August had been cancelled due to concerns over potential increased coronavirus transmission.

- Russian scientific researchers revealed that the country plans to produce 30 million doses of a COVID-19 vaccine domestically in 2020, with the possibility of manufacturing a further 170 million doses abroad. This attracted criticism from governments in the US, Canada, and the UK, who claimed that state-sponsored Russian cyber-attacks had been carried out on research institutions in their respective countries to attempt to gain information relating to coronavirus vaccine trials, although the Russian government strongly denied the allegations.
- British Health Secretary Matt Hancock announced an easing of coronavirus lockdown restrictions in the city of Leicester due to a decrease in cases. Under the new restrictions, non-essential retail outlets, schools, and nurseries will be permitted to reopen from 24 July, although bars and restaurants will remain closed; the ban on social gatherings of more than six people was also maintained, as well as bans on non-essential travel.
- A spokesperson for the Jordanian Government Amjad Adaileh, announced that commercial flights from Queen Alia International Airport will resume from August to countries on an internationally agreed safe travel list.
- Authorities in the United Arab Emirates announced that trials of a potential COVID-19 vaccine being developed jointly by the China National Pharmaceutical Group, the UAE's Ministry of Health, and the private company G42 Healthcare had entered the third phase, involving 15,000 volunteers, the first such trials to be carried out worldwide.
- President of the International Olympic Committee Thomas Bach announced that the 2022 Summer Youth Olympics, scheduled to be held in the Senegalese capital of Dakar, will

be postponed to 2026 due to the postponement of several international sporting events and the economic consequences of the coronavirus pandemic.

- Health workers in Zimbabwe issued a two weeks' strike notice to the country's government due to low wages and the lack of protective equipment needed to treat coronavirus patients safely.

17 July

- India surpasses 1 million total cases, with more than 25,000 deaths.
- Malaysia has reported 18 new cases, bringing the total to 8,755. Three have recovered, bringing the total number of recoveries to 8,541. There are 92 active cases, with three in intensive care and one on ventilator assistance. The death toll remains at 122.
- New Zealand has reported one new case, bringing the total number of cases to 1,549 (1,199 confirmed and 350 probable). Seven people recovered, bringing the total number of recovered to 1,506. There are 21 active cases, while the death toll remains at 22.
- Singapore has reported 327 new cases, bringing the total to 47,453. In addition, a patient was later confirmed to have COVID-19 after she died, which was caused by brain bleeding.
- Ukraine has reported 809 new cases and 11 new deaths, bringing the total numbers to 57,264 and 1,456, respectively; a total of 29,769 patients have recovered.
- Brazil tops 2 million cases

- Prime Minister Boris Johnson announces a further easing of lockdown restrictions for England, with plans for a "significant return to normality" by Christmas. The new rules allow people to use public transport for non-essential journeys with immediate effect, while employers will have more discretion over their workplaces from 1 August. From 18 July, local authorities will have the power to enforce local shutdowns.
- Johnson announces an extra £3bn for the NHS in England to help prepare for a possible second wave of COVID-19 over the coming winter.
- Johnson announces a pilot scheme for a return to spectator sports, with a view to a full return by 1 October. The 2020 World Snooker Championship and the Glorious Goodwood Festival are among the first two sporting events to be part of the pilot. A pilot scheme is also announced to return to indoor performances with socially distanced audiences at theatres, music, and performance venues, with a view to a full return in August.
- Health Secretary Matt Hancock calls for a review of the way COVID-19 deaths are recorded in England after Public Health England confirms it records deaths as COVID related even if the death occurs several months after someone has tested positive for the virus; the other Home Nations do not record a death as COVID related if it occurs more than 28 days after a positive test.
- Rochdale introduces extra social distancing precautions to avoid full lockdown following a rise in COVID-19 cases in the area.

- Princess Beatrice marries Edoardo Mapelli Mozzi at Windsor Castle in a private ceremony attended by the Queen and close family. The wedding has been postponed from 29 May due to the COVID-19 pandemic.
- The Queen knights captain Sir Tom Moore in a ceremony at Windsor Castle.
- British Airways announces plans to retire its entire fleet of Boeing 747s four years ahead of schedule following a downturn in travel precipitated by the COVID-19 outbreak.
- Indian pharmaceutical company Cadila Healthcare announced that late-stage trials of the company's possible COVID-19 vaccine are due to be completed in March 2021, with the potential to produce 100 million doses of the vaccine every year.
- Health authorities in the Pakistani province of Sindh extended the lockdown there until at least 15 August in response to surging coronavirus cases, with most non-essential businesses remaining closed, and residents advised to maintain a social distance of three feet and wear a face mask in all public spaces.
- Canadian Prime Minister Justin Trudeau revealed further details about the Canadian government's $14 billion economic recovery programme to restart the economy after the coronavirus pandemic. Measures included in the programme include contact tracing, providing appropriate PPE to healthcare workers, assisting financially struggling municipalities to pay operating costs, and improving long-term social care for the elderly.
- United States Secretary of the Treasury Steven Mnuchin stated that policymakers should consider blanket loan

forgiveness for smaller businesses that received funding from the Paycheck Protection Program. Additional funds could be made available, with businesses badly affected potentially entitled to a second emergency loan.

- Governor of Georgia Brian Kemp announced that he would be suing authorities in the city of Atlanta after Mayor Keisha Lance Bottoms attempted to introduce legislation requiring residents to wear face masks in public spaces; Kemp claims that city officials do not have the authority to make such a decision.
- Australian Prime Minister Scott Morrison announced a 400 million Australian dollar funding programme to provide cash grants to international film studios, with the aim of encouraging companies to work in Australia over seven years, with an estimated AU$3 billion in foreign expenditure and 8,000 jobs predicted to be created under the scheme.
- In China, the capital of the Xinjiang province Ürümqi cancelled more than 600 flights from Ürümqi Diwopu International Airport after the first case in over five months was confirmed in the province, sparking fears of a potential new wave of infections. Subway services in the city were also suspended.
- The World Health Organization announced that the team of international experts tasked with studying the spread of COVID-19 from China will be delayed to the end of July.
- Austrian Chancellor Sebastian Kurz announced that his government rejected the economic recovery programme proposed by the European Union, arguing that there should not be a long-term debt union.

- Leaders from the 27 member states of the European Union met in Brussels to discuss the proposed coronavirus economic recovery programme, which aims to disburse 750 billion euros as part of a long-term recovery plan, with all payments expected to last until 2026. . However, Czech Prime Minister Andrej Babiš later stated that the EU was no closer to reaching an agreement and that views on the proposal were widely varied.
- Authorities in Israel imposed a weekend lockdown from 17 to 19 July, with non-essential shops, zoos, museums, and leisure facilities all instructed to close. However, the government reiterated that it was not a stay-at-home order. Russian pharmaceutical company R-Pharm revealed that it had reached an agreement with AstraZeneca and the University of Oxford to manufacture the potential COVID-19 vaccine being developed by the two companies.
- Catalan Health Minister Alba Vergés urged four million residents of the Barcelona metropolitan area to stay at home as a result of a rise in coronavirus cases. All non-essential travel was advised against, with entertainment venues including cinemas and theatres being forced to close, restaurants operating at a significantly reduced capacity, and the social gathering limit to ten people.
- British Prime Minister Boris Johnson announced that fans could possibly return to sports stadiums by October, with a number of pilots schemed scheduled to take place from the end of July; these pilot schemes were later revealed to be held at two country cricket matches from 27 to 26 July, the 2020 World Snooker Championship from 31 July to 16 August, and the Goodwood horse racing festival on 1 August. All stadiums will be expected to follow strict hygiene

measures, including providing hand sanitising stations and implementing social distancing. Johnson also revealed an additional £3 billion in funding to the National Health Service to prepare for a possible second wave of coronavirus infections, with testing capacity scheduled to be increased to 500,000 a day by the end of October.

- The national airline of the United Kingdom, British Airways, announced that all of the company's Boeing 747 planes, equivalent to ten percent of the company's entire fleet, will be retired with immediate effect due to the economic consequences of the coronavirus pandemic.
- The World Food Programme and Food and Agriculture Organization jointly warned that hunger threatened "to soar to devastating levels in 25 countries in the coming months", pushing the world poorest "closer to the abyss" of famine.
- United Nations Secretary-General António Guterres, speaking during the High-Level Segment of the United Nations Economic and Social Council (ECOSOC) session to review progress towards achieving the United Nations Sustainable Development Agenda for 2030, stated that COVID-19 highlighted the need for "renewed, inclusive multilateralism" and leadership by ECOSOC, the UN's main body for deliberative and innovative strategizing.
- Commercial flights between Iran and the United Arab Emirates resumed after an Emirates plane flew from Dubai to Tehran.

18 July

- Malaysia has reported nine new cases, bringing the total to 8,764. There are 96 cases, with one case admitted to intensive care. Five cases have recovered, bringing the total to 8,546. The death toll remains at 122.
- New Zealand has reported one new case, bringing the number of cases to 1,550 (1,200 confirmed and 350 probable). There are 22 active cases, while the number of recovered remains are 1,506, and the death toll stands at 22.
- Singapore has reported 202 new cases, bringing the total to 47,655.
- Ukraine has reported 847 new cases and 21 new deaths, bringing the total numbers to 58,111 and 1,477, respectively; a total of 30,525 patients have recovered.
- Andrei Kelin, Russia's ambassador to the UK, rejects allegations that Russian intelligence agents tried to steal coronavirus vaccine research information.
- Local authorities in England get new powers to close shops and outdoor public spaces and cancel events to control COVID-19.
- The 2020 Indianapolis 500 was delayed until August of the same year.
- Authorities in Azerbaijan announced that coronavirus lockdown restrictions will be extended to August 31 after a further surge in cases. It was stated that people in urban areas, including the capital Baku, must obtain special permission to leave their homes between July 20 and August 5, with non-essential businesses including shopping centres,

restaurants, and entertainment facilities all remaining closed; beauty salons were given permission to reopen.

- Leaders of member states of the European Union reconvened in Brussels to discuss the proposed 750 billion euro economic recovery plan. Officials stated that several wealthy northern countries had expressed concern over access to the recovery fund; several leaders stated that the negotiations had been challenging, with German Chancellor Angela Merkel describing them as "very, very difficult negotiations" and Polish Prime Minister Mateusz Morawiecki stating that it is "highly probable" that a deal will not be reached by Sunday.
- Greek authorities extended the coronavirus lockdown in the country's migrant camps to August 2 in order to prevent the further spread of the virus.
- The British Government temporarily suspended daily reporting on new COVID-19 deaths after some scientists claimed that Public Health England has been over-reporting new deaths. Also, in the UK, a COVID-19 antibody test developed by the University of Oxford passed the first phase of scientific trials with over 98 percent accuracy.
- The leaders of the G20 took part in a virtual meeting hosted by the Saudi capital of Riyadh to discuss the recovery of the global economy. The G20 had previously announced a one-year debt freeze for poorer countries, although World Bank President David Malpass recommended, extending the scheme to 2022. The G20 leaders concluded the meeting by stating that a possible extension to the debt suspension scheme would be discussed further at the 2020 G20 Riyadh summit.

19 July

- Malaysia has reported 15 new cases (11 community transmissions and four imported), bringing the total to 8,779. There are 103 active cases, with two in intensive care and one on ventilator support. One new death was reported, bringing the death toll to 123.
- New Zealand has reported three new cases, bringing the total number of cases to 1,553 (1,203 confirmed and 350 probable). There are 25 active cases, while the number of recovered remains is 1,506, and the death toll stands at 22.
- Singapore has reported 257 new cases, bringing the total to 47,912.
- Ukraine has reported 731 new cases and 8 new deaths, bringing the total numbers to 58,842 and 1,485, respectively; a total of 30,879 patients have recovered.
- Prime Minister Boris Johnson tells *The Sunday Telegraph* he does not believe it will be necessary to impose a second nationwide lockdown in the event of a spike in COVID-19 cases, comparing the option to a "nuclear deterrent."
- Robert Buckland, the Secretary of State for Justice, announces the creation of ten temporary courts in England and Wales to deal with a backlog of legal cases brought about by the pandemic.
- The United Nations highlighted the plight of hundreds of thousands of seafarers stranded at sea, some for over a year, due to COVID-19 travel restrictions.
- Iran's Civil Aviation Organisation announced that Turkish authorities suspended flights to and from the country due to new coronavirus outbreaks in Iran.

- The Iranian Health Ministry confirmed the country's number of cases to be significantly lower than the 25 million previously suggested by President Hassan Rouhani.
- President of Chile Sebastian Piñera revealed his government's plan to gradually reopen the country's economy after a sustained fall in daily infections. Officials stated that the programme will take place for five weeks, although any progress would be subject to epidemiological data and the capacity of the country's healthcare system.
- President of El Salvador Nayib Bukele announced that the country will move into the second phase of reopening after the coronavirus pandemic, with manufacturing industries and public transport scheduled to reopen on July 21.
- Nigerian Foreign Minister Geoffrey Onyeama announced that he would be self-isolating after testing positive for COVID-19, becoming the first member of the Nigerian Cabinet to do so.
- The United Nations issued an urgent appeal to member states to provide almost $300 million in financial aid to Sudan to assist the country in fighting the coronavirus pandemic and dealing with the economic consequences.
- Leaders of the member states of the European Union did not reach an agreement on proposed economic recovery grants after the third day of talks in Brussels. It was reported that the main disagreements lie with the size of the grants, with several countries, led by the Netherlands, stating that 350 billion euros should be the maximum amount, whilst others stated that 400 billion euros should be the minimum amount.

- French Health Minister Olivier Véran announced that from July 20, there will be a fine of 135 euros for people caught without a face mask in indoor public spaces.
- Minister-President of the German state of Bavaria Markus Söder stated that free coronavirus tests will soon be provided for returning passengers at all airports in the state.
- Health officials in the Spanish autonomous community of Catalonia strongly advised residents to stay at home in the municipalities of Figueres, Vilafant, and Sant Feliu de Llobregat after a surge in coronavirus cases. Although no mandatory lockdown was imposed, new restrictions included reducing the social gathering limit to ten people and restaurants were operating at a 50 percent capacity, with strict social distancing measures in place. Authorities in Barcelona also announced that law enforcement officers will limit access to the city's beaches as a result of rising cases in the city and its surrounding areas.
- Premier of the Australian state of Victoria, Daniel Andrews, announced that it will now be mandatory for the public to wear face masks in public areas due to the rising coronavirus cases in the state, with fines of up to 200 Australian dollars if caught without one.
- Health authorities in the Chinese province of Xinjiang declared the capital Ürümqi and the surrounding area to be in a "wartime situation" due to the recent outbreak of coronavirus infections in the city. Several restrictions were introduced, including a ban on visits to different households and mass COVID-19 screening in public buildings; authorities also urged residents of Ürümqi not to leave the city for non-essential reasons.

- Chief Executive of Hong Kong Carrie Lam announced a tightening of coronavirus restrictions in Hong Kong due to the surging daily infections in the city. All non-essential civil servants were instructed to work from home. Face masks were made mandatory in all indoor public areas, with non-essential leisure businesses including gyms and theme parks remaining closed for an additional week.

20 July

- Malaysia has reported 21 new cases. Two patients were discharged, bringing the total number of recovered to 8,555. There are 122 active cases, with three in intensive care and one needing ventilator assistance.
- New Zealand has reported one new case, bringing the total number to 1,554 (1,204 confirmed and 350 probable). There are 26 active cases, while the number of recovered remains 1,506, and the death toll stands at 22.
- Singapore has reported 123 new cases, bringing the total to 48,035.
- Ukraine has reported 651 new cases and 13 new deaths, bringing the total numbers to 59,493 and 1,498, respectively; a total of 31,439 patients have recovered.
- The UK has signed a deal for 90 million doses of promising vaccines being developed jointly by the pharmaceutical companies BioNTech and Pfizer and by Valneva. This is in addition to the 100 million doses being developed by the University of Oxford and AstraZeneca.
- Preliminary results of clinical trials of a drug developed by Southampton-based biotech firm Synairgen that uses the protein interferon beta have shown promising signs. The

treatment involves a patient inhaling the protein produced by the body to fight viral infections into the lungs using a nebuliser in order to encourage an immune response.

- Clinical trials of the vaccine developed by the University of Oxford on 1,077 patients show that it appears safe and trains the immune system to produce COVID-19 antibodies.
- Boris Johnson says he is confident but not "100% confident" a vaccine will be available in 2020.
- The UK Government is investing £14m in two factories at Port Talbot, South Wales, and Blackburn, Lancashire, to produce a million high-quality face coverings per week.
- High Street retailer Marks & Spencer announces 950 job losses as a result of the continuing economic impact of the pandemic.
- Authorities in Saudi Arabia announced that the annual Hajj pilgrimage to Mecca will begin on July 29, with social distancing guidelines in place and a heavily reduced capacity.
- Bahamian Prime Minister Hubert Minnis announced that the country's borders will be closed to international flights and ships from July 22; Minnis stated that the UK, USA, and Canada would be exempt from the restrictions.
- Despite announcing yesterday that El Salvador would move into the second phase of reopening after the COVID-19 pandemic, President Nayib Bukele postponed all further reopening plans for the foreseeable future after discussions with health experts.
- United States President Donald Trump announced that the government's daily coronavirus briefings will resume this week.

- Cinemas in several "low-risk" Chinese cities were permitted to reopen at 30 percent capacity, with mandatory temperatures checks on arrival and the requirement for customers and staff to wear face masks; the sale of refreshments was also prohibited. Some cities, including the capital Beijing, kept their cinemas closed instead of allowing local authorities to decide whether or not to reopen them.
- Several major international banking companies in Hong Kong announced that they would temporarily close some branches in the city due to a surge in domestically transmitted coronavirus cases. Banks closing some services included HSBC, Bank of China, Standard Chartered, and Bank of East Asia.
- Malaysian Prime Minister Muhyiddin Yassin has announced that the Malaysian Government is considering making face masks compulsory following the emergence of 13 clusters after the Government relaxed lockdown restrictions on movement and businesses in June 2020.
- With Latin America now being the epicentre of the pandemic, the World Health Organization expressed concern at COVID-19's impact on indigenous people in the Americas.
- Danish Business Minister Simon Kollerup stated that merchant sailors stranded at sea during the coronavirus pandemic will be permitted to dock at Danish ports due to a sustained drop in cases in the country.
- Organisers of the 2020 Ballon d'Or cancelled the award for the first time in its 64-year history due to the impact of coronavirus on the sporting industry.
- A spokesperson for the Greek government announced that tighter restrictions will be introduced to control the movement

of international seasonal workers, with any agricultural workers leaving the country before August 4 not able to return until further notice. It was also announced that land entry into Greece will be limited to six northern border crossings to control any possible imported cases.

- Health authorities in the United Kingdom revealed that the government has purchased 90 million doses of potential COVID-19 vaccines from several pharmaceutical companies, including Pfizer, Valneva SE, and BioNTech. The British government has already secured 100 million doses of a potential vaccine developed by AstraZeneca.

21 July

- Malaysia has reported 15 new cases, bringing the total number to 8,815 cases. There were seven recoveries, bringing the total number of recoveries to 8,562. There are 130 active cases, with four in intensive care and one on respirator support. The death toll remains at 123.
- New Zealand has reported one new case, bringing the total number to 1,555 (1,205 confirmed and 350 probable). There are 27 active cases while the number of recovered remains 15, 06, and the death toll stands at 22.
- Singapore has reported 399 new cases, bringing the total to 48,434.
- Ukraine has reported 673 new cases and 20 new deaths, bringing the total numbers to 60,166 and 1,518, respectively; a total of 32,199 patients have recovered.
- Chancellor Rishi Sunak announces that 900,000 public sector workers, including doctors and teachers, will get an above-inflation pay rise of 3.1% to acknowledge the important role they have played during the pandemic.

- Health experts, including Wellcome Trust director Professor Sir Jeremy Farrar, tell the House of Commons Health Committee that the UK is likely to live with COVID-19 for many years even with a vaccine.
- Regional Director for the Americas at the World Health Organization Carissa Etienne stated that the coronavirus pandemic is still rapidly spreading through in the Americas and is showing "no signs of slowing down."
- Advanced trials of a potential COVID-19 vaccine being developed by Chinese Biopharmaceutical Company Sinovac Biotech and the Instituto Butantan began in the Brazilian state of São Paulo, involving around 900 volunteers employed in the healthcare sector. Brazilian Health Minister Eduardo Pazuello also revealed that the government was in discussions with American pharmaceutical company Moderna to potentially prioritising purchasing a possible COVID-19 vaccine being developed by the company.
- United States Minority Senate Leader Chuck Schumer urged leaders of the Republican Party to present details for further coronavirus legislation in the United States Congress.
- Authorities in Oman announced that from July 25 to August 8, all travel between the country's provinces will be suspended. A night-time curfew will be imposed, during which all public spaces must close to prevent the transmission of coronavirus.
- South Africa's Labour Minister Thulas Nxesi and Minister of Mineral Resources Gwede Mantashe were admitted separately to the hospital after testing positive for coronavirus over a week ago.

- President of Zimbabwe Emmerson Mnangagwa announced that a night-time curfew will be enforced from July 22 to slow the spread of coronavirus in the country.
- Health authorities in the Chinese province of Xinjiang announced that free coronavirus tests will be provided to the 3.5 million residents of the capital Ürümqi after a recent outbreak of cases there. The Civil Aviation Administration of China also announced that passengers on international flights to China must provide evidence of a negative COVID-19 test result taken at most five days before departure to be allowed to board the plane.
- The New Zealand Health Minister Chris Hipkins announced that the Government would be investing NZ$302 million into various health services over the next two years, including the National Close Contact Service, the National Immunisation Solution, telehealth services, and purchasing more ventilators, respiratory equipment, and personal protective equipment supplies.
- The United Nation's Special Coordinator for the Middle East Peace Process warned that cooperation between Israelis and Palestinians on the COVID-19 pandemic was breaking down, "putting human lives at risk."
- The International Organization for Migration warned that fear of the COVID-19 pandemic was causing fresh displacement in war-torn Yemen.
- Authorities in Nepal announced that international flights to and from the country will resume on August 17 after being suspended during the coronavirus pandemic.
- Austrian Chancellor Sebastian Kurz reintroduced legislation mandating the wearing of face coverings in public spaces,

including supermarkets and banks, as a result of a surge in coronavirus infections in the country.

- President of the European Council Charles Michel announced that leaders of the European Union had reached an agreement over a coronavirus economic recovery fund dubbed Next Generation EU after four days of negotiations. Under the scheme, 750 billion euros of joint debt will be issued to assist the recovery of the economies of all member states, comprising 390 billion euros of grants and 360 billion euros of low-interest loans. A long-term recovery fund will also provide economic aid from 2021 to 2027.
- Polish Education Minister Dariusz Piontkowski stated that the government is working to fully reopen schools at the start of the academic year in September and is working on legislation to ensure the safety of students and staff.
- The Russian Finance Ministry revealed plans to cut government spending by up to 10 percent (a total of $65 billion) between 2021 and 2023 as a result of increased spending during the coronavirus pandemic, with the Russian GDP predicted to decrease by up to 5 percent in 2020.
- Spanish Foreign Affairs Minister Arancha González Laya announced that the Spanish government will provide 1.7 billion euros in aid to developing countries to assist them in fighting the COVID-19 pandemic.
- Sarah Gilbert, the lead researcher of the potential COVID-19 vaccine being developed by the University of Oxford and AstraZeneca, stated that the vaccine could possibly be available for purchase by the end of the year after the first stages of clinical trials showed that the vaccine initiated an immune response in volunteers.

22 July

- Malaysia has reported 16 new cases, bringing the total number to 8,831. Five active cases remain in intensive care while one requires a ventilator. There have been four recoveries.
- New Zealand has reported no new cases, with the number of active cases staying at 27 and the total number 1,555 (1,205 confirmed and 350 probable). There have been a total of 1,506 recoveries, and the death toll stands at 22.
- Singapore has reported 310 new cases, bringing the total to 48,744.
- Ukraine has reported 829 new cases and 16 new deaths, bringing the total numbers to 60,995 and 1,534, respectively; a total of 33,172 patients have recovered.
- Figures released by the Home Office reveal that a backlog of 400,000 passport applications have accumulated due to disruption caused by the COVID-19 pandemic.
- An Office for National Statistics report has concluded that a majority of children have struggled with learning at home during the lockdown.
- Fitness coach Joe Wicks presents his final online PE with Joe's exercise class after leading the daily sessions for the past 18 weeks.
- Organisers of the holy Hindu pilgrimage to Amarnath Temple cancelled the event due to the surging coronavirus cases in the Indian-controlled territory of Kashmir.
- Officials in Thailand stated that the country's state of emergency imposed to control the coronavirus pandemic will be extended to the end of August, despite the Thai government not reporting a domestically transmitted case in

almost two months. Taweesin Visanuyothin, a spokesperson for the Thai Health Ministry, stated that business executives, migrant labourers, film crews, and medical tourists will be gradually permitted to travel to the country in an attempt to recover some economic losses; all arriving travellers will be tested for COVID-19 on arrival and must undergo a mandatory 14-day quarantine.

23 July

- Face masks became mandatory in the Australian city of Melbourne after surging coronavirus cases in the state of Victoria. The Victoria State Government announced that workers who do not have sick leave will be able to apply for a payment of 300 Australian dollars. At the same time, they await a COVID-19 test result after reports suggested that recent outbreaks could be attributed to employees not taking time off work to wait for results.
- Hong Kong Secretary for Food and Health Sophia Chan announced that face masks will be mandatory on public transport and in indoor spaces, as well as transport hubs, with immediate effect until August 5 due to recent outbreaks of the virus in Hong Kong. Chan also urged residents to only travel for essential reasons.
- The Japanese Health Ministry approved the use of dexamethasone to treat moderate or advanced cases of COVID-19 after trials showed that the drug significantly reduced the mortality rate.
- President of the Democratic Republic of the Congo Félix Tshisekedi lifted the country's health emergency imposed to control the coronavirus outbreak due to a sustained drop in new deaths. Tshisekedi revealed a three-stage plan to

reopen the country's schools, businesses, and international borders; from July 23, non-essential businesses including banks and restaurants will be permitted to reopen, as well as social gatherings and public transport.

- Managers at restaurants and bars in South Africa urged the government to lift coronavirus restrictions preventing the sale of alcohol after 9 pm, claiming that such services provide vital sources of income for businesses.
- Independent United Nations, human rights experts, called for Iran to urgently release human rights activist Narges Mohammadi, reportedly ill with COVID-19 symptoms, together with other arbitrarily detained individuals, "before it is too late."
- Spanish Tourism Minister Reyes Maroto stated that the France-Spain border should stay open as the recent outbreaks of coronavirus in Catalonia come under control.
- Organisers of the Nobel Prizes cancelled the traditional banquet, scheduled to be held in December at Stockholm City Hall, for the first time since 1956 due to public health concerns relating to the pandemic.
- Health authorities in Switzerland expanded the country's coronavirus watch list to include a total of 42 countries; travellers arriving from these countries are required to undergo a mandatory 14-day quarantine upon entry to Switzerland or receive a fine of 10,000 Swiss francs. The new additions to the list included Bosnia & Herzegovina, Costa Rica, Ecuador, El Salvador, eSwatini, Guatemala, Kazakhstan, Kyrgyzstan, Luxembourg, the Maldives, Mexico, Montenegro, Suriname, and the United Arab Emirates. Sweden and Belarus were removed from the list.

- President of Ukraine Volodymyr Zelensky announced that tourists arriving in the country from Australia, New Zealand, and several Arab states will no longer require a visa in an attempt to increase tourism after the COVID-19 pandemic.
- The National Football League announced that all spectators will be required to wear face masks when the season resumes in September to reduce the risk of coronavirus transmission.
- Mayor of Washington, D.C. Muriel Bowser announced that face masks will be made compulsory in all areas outside of the home due to a recent rise in cases in the city, with authorities citing the effectiveness of similar orders elsewhere in reducing transmission of the virus. Exceptions to the rule include children under three, exercising at a suitable distance from others, and working alone in an office. This comes as President Donald Trump urged Americans to wear face masks in public, the first time he has advocated such a measure.
- The United States Department of Health and Human Services announced that the U.S. government will pay the pharmaceutical companies Pfizer and BioNTech $1.95 billion to produce an initial order of 100 million doses of a potential COVID-19 vaccine, with the government then able to acquire an additional 500 million doses.
- The Egyptian government extended the permitted operating hours for restaurants to midnight and increased the permitted capacity to 50 percent. The operating hours for shops were extended to 10 pm; both pieces of legislation will come into effect from July 26.

- The Qatari government announced that the country's borders will reopen to international travellers from August 1 to further ease coronavirus lockdown restrictions. All arriving travellers from a list of 40 countries deemed to be low-risk will be required to take a COVID-19 test at the airport and undergo a mandatory quarantine for a week whilst awaiting the result; anybody testing positive will be transferred to a secure government facility to self-isolate.

24 July

- Malaysia has reported nine new cases, bringing the total to 8,840. There are 143 active cases, with five in intensive care and two needing ventilation assistance. Eight have recovered, bringing the total number of recovered to 8,574. The death toll remains at 123.
- New Zealand has reported five new recoveries, bringing the active number of cases to 22 and the number of recovered to 1,511. There were no new cases, with the total number remaining at 1,555 (1,205 confirmed and 350 probable). The death toll remains at 22.
- Singapore has reported 354 new cases, bringing the total to 49,098.
- Ukraine has reported 856 new cases and 17 new deaths, bringing the total numbers to 61,851 and 1,551, respectively; a total of 34,000 patients have recovered.
- During a visit to Scotland to mark the first year of taking office as Prime Minister, Boris Johnson says that the response to the COVID-19 pandemic proves the "sheer might" and "merits of the union."

- A report published by the House of Commons Public Accounts Committee criticises the UK government for its "astonishing" failure to plan for the economic impact of the COVID-19 pandemic.
- The House of Commons Culture Select Committee criticises the government for being too slow to respond to what it describes as the "existential threat" faced by live theatre, music, and other culture because of the effects of the COVID-19 pandemic.
- Vacuum cleaner manufacturer Dyson announces the loss of 900 jobs, 600 of them in the UK, as a result of the financial impact of the COVID-19 pandemic.
- Northern Ireland's Department of Health confirms the release of Northern Ireland's contact-tracing app, StopCOVID NI, for as early as 29 July. Northern Ireland is the first part of the UK to launch a contact-tracing app.
- The United Nations High-level Advisory Board on Economic and Social Affairs released the report Recover Better: Economic and Social Challenges and Opportunities, calling for “an adjusted approach” to economic development and global solidarity in response to the worst recession in decades and the first rise in global poverty since 1998.
- The United Nations Secretary-General highlighted that the pandemic could provide a new opportunity to resolve long-standing conflicts and address structural problems in the Arab world.
- The incoming United Nations ECOSOC President, Ambassador Munir Akram of Pakistan, outlined a triple focus on the pandemic, the SDGs, and climate action.

- In September, the United Nations confirmed that it would host its first 'virtual' UN General Assembly.
- The Director-General of the World Health Organization urged people to play their part in preventing further spread of the pandemic, warning of no return to "the old normal" as global cases topped 15 million.
- The China National Pharmaceutical Group stated that the company's potential COVID-19 vaccine could be available for purchase by the end of the year, despite previous estimates of vaccine trials not being completed until 2021. Researchers stated that clinical trials of the potential vaccine should be completed within three months.
- Authorities in Papua New Guinea asked the World Health Organization to deploy an emergency medical team to assist the country in fighting the coronavirus pandemic after almost twenty of the country's thirty cases were reported within a week.
- Authorities in the Philippines reimposed a ban on non-essential domestically and internationally due to complications with health insurance and surging infection rates in many parts of the world.
- The Bank of Korea reported that South Korea's gross domestic product (GDP) contracted by 3.3 percent in the second fiscal quarter between April and June, making it the steepest decline since 1998. The country's vital exports industry also declined by a record 16.6 percent.
- The African Development Bank announced an aid package worth $285 million to assist several countries in the Sahel region in fighting the pandemic. Under the scheme, Niger will receive $110 million, Burkina Faso $55 million, Mali $50

million in loans and grants, Chad will receive $60 million, and Mauritania $10 million in grants.

- South African President Cyril Ramaphosa announced that all public schools in the country will close from July 27 for four weeks to limit coronavirus transmission, as the number of confirmed cases in South Africa passed 400,000. Ramaphosa also revealed a 500 billion rand ($30 billion) economic support package to fund the healthcare sector fighting the pandemic.
- Israeli Prime Minister Benjamin Netanyahu appointed Ronni Gamzu, the director of the Tel Aviv Sourasky Medical Center, as the country's National Coronavirus Project Manager; Gamzu will be responsible for coordinating the Israeli government's response to the pandemic.
- The Dutch Museum Association urged Prime Minister Mark Rutte to provide the country's arts industry with vital economic support as a result of months of closures during the COVID-19 pandemic, with a large number of smaller businesses warning that they could potentially go bankrupt without further support from the Dutch government.
- Statistics Sweden revealed that Sweden's unemployment rate reached 9.4 percent in June as a direct result of the economic consequences of the coronavirus pandemic, the highest level of unemployment recorded in the country since 1998. 557,000 people were recorded as being unemployed, 150,000 higher than at the same time in 2019.
- Malaysian Senior Minister Ismail Sabri Yaakob has announced that it will be compulsory to wear face masks in public spaces such as markets and public transportation from 1 August. Violators may face an RM1, 000 (US$235 fine).

- Bolivia's Plurinational Electoral Organ postponed the country's general election, scheduled to be taking place in early September, to October 18 as a result of restrictions imposed to fight the coronavirus pandemic and experts predicting that the virus will spike in Bolivia in August or September.
- The Chilean Parliament passed legislation allowing citizens to withdraw up to 10 percent of their pension savings to reduce the economic consequences of the coronavirus pandemic. However, President Sebastian Piñera must sign it into effect.
- Mexican Foreign Affairs Minister Marcelo Ebrard stated that Chinese officials offered a $1 billion loan to Latin America and the Caribbean to provide any potential COVID-19 vaccine developed by a Chinese company.
- The Walt Disney Company postponed the debuts of several films due to the coronavirus pandemic. The release of the live-action version of Mulan was postponed indefinitely, and the releases of Avatar 2 and a new Star Wars film were postponed to December 2022 and December 2023, respectively.
- The United States Department of Labor revealed that over 1.4 million American citizens applied for unemployment benefits in the last week, an increase on the figure reported last week, despite several weeks of decreasing numbers.
- The 66th Annual Art in the Park (the major fundraiser for the Boise Art Museum, scheduled to be held in September) was cancelled as an in-person event and shifted to the virtual realm. Two major Jehovah's Witnesses conventions were also cancelled, as was the Veteran's Day Parade.

- The Kuwaiti government announced that the country's curfew will be adjusted to be in place from 9 pm to 3 am and will be reviewed after the Eid al-Adha festival; it was also announced that the third phase of reopening after the pandemic will begin on July 28. Under the new restrictions, hotels and places of worship will be permitted to reopen, and taxi drivers will also be allowed to resume operations.
- Newly released data from the World Health Organization highlighted that the countries of Qatar and Bahrain have the highest per capita rates of coronavirus infection anywhere in the world.

25 July

- The Australian state of Victoria has reported 300 new cases and six new deaths in the past 24 hours. In addition, 447 cases were linked to aged care facilities in that state.
- Malaysia has reported 21 new cases, bringing the total to 8,861. There are 161 active cases, with five in intensive care and two on ventilator assistance. Three patients have recovered, bringing the total number of recovered to 8,577. The death toll remains at 123.
- New Zealand has reported one new case, bringing the total number of cases to 1,556 (1,206 confirmed and 350 probable). There have been two cases, bringing the total number of recovered to 1,513. There are 21 active cases.
- Singapore has reported 277 new cases, bringing the total to 49,375.
- Ukraine has reported 972 new cases and 20 new deaths, bringing the total numbers to 62,823 and 1,571, respectively; a total of 34,886 patients have recovered.

- The United States surpasses 4 million cases
- In an interview with BBC political editor Laura Kuenssberg, Prime Minister Boris Johnson says that the UK government did not understand the nature of coronavirus at the beginning of the pandemic and could have done things differently. He also says there are "open questions" about whether lockdown was implemented too late.
- Face coverings have become compulsory in shops and most other enclosed public places in England.
- The list of countries where travellers do not have to quarantine when arriving in England is updated, adding Estonia, Latvia, Slovakia, Slovenia, and St Vincent and the Grenadines; travellers from Portugal must still isolate for 14 days.
- Office for National Statistics figures show that retail sales increased almost to pre-lockdown levels in June, rising 13.9% compared to May.
- The UN human rights office (OHCHR) reminded authorities in Zimbabwe that the coronavirus pandemic should not be used as "an excuse to clamp down on fundamental freedoms."
- The health ministry of Senegal announced that four new coronavirus testing centres will be constructed in the capital Dakar to increase the testing capacity for arriving travellers.
- Authorities in the Chinese coastal city of Dalian placed the city into a "war-time mode" to contain a recent outbreak of COVID-19 cases linked to a seafood factory. New restrictions imposed by the government include mandatory tests for anybody travelling on the city's subway system, nurseries being forced to close, and the potential for some

communities to be placed under a lockdown if authorities see no improvement in the situation.

- The Chinese Civil Aviation Authority revealed that daily commercial flights had increased to approximately 80 percent of pre-COVID levels as a result of authorities lifting restrictions imposed on the aviation industry in recent months.
- Bulgarian Prime Minister Boyko Borisov entered a period of self-isolation after a senior government official tested positive for COVID-19.
- French Prime Minister Jean Castex advised French citizens not to travel to the Spanish autonomous community of Catalonia after a surge of cases in the region and also announced that there will be increased controls at French borders with travellers arriving from some countries having to undergo mandatory COVID-19 tests.
- German Health Minister Jens Spahn announced that travellers arriving from countries deemed to have high rates of coronavirus transmission might be required to take a mandatory COVID-19 test at the airport or undergo a 14-day quarantine.
- Italian Health Minister Roberto Speranza announced that any travellers arriving in Italy from Bulgaria and Romania would be required to enter a mandatory quarantine to prevent the importation of any COVID-19 cases.
- Norwegian health authorities announced that any travellers arriving in the country from Spain will be required to enter a mandatory 10-day quarantine as a result of surging cases there. It was also announced that free travel will resume

between Norway and the Swedish regions of Kalmar, Örebro, Östergötland, and Värmland.

- Chilean Health Minister Enrique Paris announced an easing of coronavirus lockdown restrictions in the capital city of Santiago. Under the new restrictions, residents of the city's least densely populated suburbs will be permitted to gather in small groups and leave their homes without permission from authorities.
- The Nicaraguan Government announced that citizens returning to the country will not be allowed to enter without proof of a negative coronavirus test result in the last 72 hours, which resulted in several hundred Nicaraguan travellers becoming stranded at the Costa Rica-Nicaragua border.
- Mayor of Washington, D.C. Muriel Bowser announced that from July 27, travellers arriving into Washington, D.C. for non-essential reasons from any area deemed to be a coronavirus hotspot must enter a mandatory 14-day quarantine to reduce the risk of transmission. However, the neighbouring states of Maryland and Virginia were excluded from the restrictions. Despite the increasing restrictions, the US National Zoological Park in Washington, D.C., reopened with various coronavirus measures in place. Visitors must pre-book tickets, with a reduced capacity, and face masks are compulsory for both visitors and staff; social distancing measures were also introduced, with some areas of the zoo implementing a one-way system.
- Speaker of the United States House of Representatives Nancy Pelosi stated that she was not considering an extension to the enhanced unemployment benefits scheme, scheduled to end on July 31.

- White House Press Secretary Kayleigh McEnany stated that President Trump aims to fully reopen all American schools at the start of the academic year despite concerns from teachers and parents about a potential increase in transmission of COVID-19.

26 July

- Malaysia has reported 23 new cases, bringing the total number to 8,884. 17 have recovered, bringing the total number of recovered to 8,594. There are 167 active cases, with three in intensive care and two on ventilator assistance. The death toll remains at 123.
- New Zealand has reported no new cases, with the number of active cases remaining 21. The total number of cases remains 1,556 (1,206 confirmed and 350 probable), the number recovered at 1,513, and the death toll 22.
- Singapore has reported 513 new cases, bringing the total to 49,888.
- Ukraine has reported 1,106 new cases and 19 new deaths, bringing the total numbers to 63,929 and 1,590, respectively; a total of 35,497 patients have recovered.
- Sahrawi Arab Democratic Republic reports its first four cases.
- Public Health England warns that being obese and overweight puts people at greater risk of severe illness or death as a result of COVID-19.
- Share prices in Synairgen are reported to have increased by 540% after news of the successful interferon-beta-based drug trial.

- Following a rise in COVID-19 cases in Spain and concerns of a second wave, the UK Government confirms travellers returning to England from Spain will be required to quarantine for 14 days from 26 July.
- Iranian President Hassan Rouhani urged the public to follow social distancing measures in order to prevent a second spike of infections in the country during the Islamic festival of Eid al-Adha, which begins at the end of July.
- Authorities in Kuwait announced that the coronavirus lockdown imposed in Farwaniya Governorate will be lifted on July 26.
- South African Trade Minister Ebrahim Patel tested positive for COVID-19, and thus he and all ministers with whom he had come into contact entered a period of self-isolation.
- The Chinese capital of Beijing partially reopened cinemas in districts with lower rates of coronavirus transmission. Under the new restrictions, all tickets must be pre-booked, social distancing must be maintained, and venues can only operate at thirty percent capacity; it was also announced that mandatory temperature screening will be enforced upon entry.
- Prime Minister of Vietnam Nguyễn Xuân Phúc signed legislation prohibiting all wildlife imports and the operation of wildlife markets after considerable scientific evidence of increased transmission involving such industries; tougher penalties for poachers will also be introduced. This comes as Vietnam recorded its first domestically transmitted case of COVID-19 in over three months.
- Chilean President Sebastián Piñera signed a law allowing citizens to withdraw up to ten percent of their pension

savings to reduce the economic consequences of the pandemic, thus bringing the law into effect.

- The Supreme Court of the United States voted to maintain legislation imposed by the state government of Nevada, which prevented more than fifty people from gathering together after a Calvary Chapel in Dayton Valley requested changes to the legislation to allow larger religious services.
- Tapan Mishra, the United Nations Resident Coordinator in Mongolia, warned of a major economic impact from the pandemic and development setback, despite its very few cases of COVID-19.
- Spanish Minister for Foreign Affairs Arancha González Laya stated that the recent localised coronavirus outbreaks in the country were under control, and affected communities had been promptly isolated. González also stated that discussions were ongoing with foreign governments to arrange travel restrictions.
- The British Government announced that travellers arriving in the country from mainland Spain will be required to enter a 14-day self-isolation due to a recent outbreak of cases in several regions. Spain had been removed from the government's list of safe countries. Thus all non-essential travel was advised against, prompting several airlines and tour operators to cancel flights.
- Malaysian Trade Minister Mohamed Azmin Ali stated that the 2020 Asia-Pacific Economic Cooperation summit could potentially go ahead in the capital Kuala Lumpur in November, despite various international travel restrictions imposed the COVID-19 pandemic.

27 July

- Malaysia has reported 13 new cases, bringing the total number of cases to 8,897. Six patients have recovered, bringing the total number of recovered to 8,600. One death was reported, bringing the death toll to 124.
- New Zealand has reported no new cases. The total number of cases remains 1,556 (1,206 confirmed and 350 probable), the number recovered at 1,513, and the death toll 22. There are 21 active cases.
- Singapore has reported 481 new cases, bringing the total to 50,369.
- Ukraine has reported 920 new cases and 15 new deaths, bringing the total numbers to 64,849 and 1,605, respectively; a total of 35,807 patients have recovered.
- The U.S.A reported 143 663 deaths.
- Foreign Secretary Dominic Raab says it was right to act quickly, following criticism of the government's short-notice decision to reimpose quarantine rules on travellers arriving from Spain.
- The UK's largest tour operator, Tui, cancels all flights from the UK to mainland Spain until 9 August
- Transport Secretary Grant Shapps, who flew out to Spain for a holiday the previous day, is caught by the change of quarantine rules.
- Indian Aviation Minister Hardeep Singh Puri revealed that over 800,000 Indian citizens had been repatriated from over fifty countries since May under the government's Vande Bharat Mission.
- Malaysian Senior Minister Ismail Sabri Yaakob announced that the federal government will limit inter-zone movement in

Sarawak, particularly around the state capital Kuchin in a bid to curb the spread of COVID-19 within that state.

- Cruise tour operator Genting Hong Kong resumed island-hopping cruises around the Taiwanese islands with several coronavirus restrictions: social distancing must be maintained at all times, increased ventilation, routine sanitisation of public areas, and all crew members were placed in a three-week quarantine with mandatory COVID-19 tests before the cruise departed.
- North Korean Supreme Leader Kim Jong-UN imposed a total coronavirus lockdown and declared a state of emergency in the border city of Kaesong over concerns of a possible outbreak in the city after authorities identified an individual expressing COVID-19 symptoms. ,. According to North Korean state media, the suspected case and all of their social contacts have been placed into quarantine.
- Health authorities in the Vietnamese city of Da Nang announced a tightening of coronavirus lockdown measures after Vietnam reported its first two domestically transmitted cases in over three months. Under the new restrictions, gatherings of more than thirty people are prohibited, and non-essential businesses, including amusement parks, bars, beauty salons, and nightclubs, were ordered to close.
- A study by the international news agency Reuters revealed for the first time that Latin America has the highest number of coronavirus cases than any other region in the world, with over 4.3 million confirmed cases.
- The United States Government announced a further $470 million in funding to the biopharmaceutical company Moderna to support the company's development of a

potential COVID-19 vaccine, particularly involving the third phase of clinical trials.

- President of Madagascar Andry Rajoelina opened a new coronavirus testing centre in the capital city of Antananarivo, able to accommodate up to 250 patients expressing severe coronavirus symptoms in response to surging cases overwhelming the country's healthcare system.
- European tour operator TUI cancelled all holiday bookings to mainland Spain up to 9 August and all bookings to the Canary Islands and the Balearic Islands up to 4 August due to international travel restrictions imposed in response to a surge in coronavirus cases in some Spanish regions.
- French health authorities announced that PCR nasal swab tests for COVID-19 will be made available for free in response to a rise in new cases recorded in the country.
- Health authorities in the Bavarian district of Dingolfing-Landau imposed a lockdown on 480 employees at a farm after a recent outbreak led to over 170 testings positive for COVID-19.
- President of the Italian region of Campania Vincenzo De Luca announced that people who do not wear a face mask in indoor areas in the city of Salerno will receive a 1,000 euro fine, with transport operators receiving powers to deny access passengers who refuse to wear a mask. It was also announced that businesses failing to comply with coronavirus restrictions imposed by the regional or national government could also be fined and be ordered to close for up to thirty days.
- Authorities in Hong Kong announced a further tightening of coronavirus restrictions in effect from July 29 after a recent

surge in cases. Under the new restrictions, social gatherings of more than two people will be prohibited, all restaurants must close indoor dining, and face masks will be made mandatory in all public spaces, both indoors and outdoors.

- Japanese Economic Minister Yasutoshi Nishimura urged business leaders to improve coronavirus preventative measures, including increasing telecommunications to encourage employees to work from home.
- Authorities in Vietnam postponed the 2020 ASEAN summit to September. They instructed over 80,000 tourists in the city of Da Nang to leave the country after a recent outbreak of domestically transmitted cases, despite not reporting any new cases in three months.

28 July

- Malaysia has reported seven new cases, bringing the total number to 8,904. There are 179 active cases, while the death toll remains at 124. One patient has recovered, bringing the total to 8,601.
- New Zealand has reported no new cases. The total number of cases remains 1,556 (1,206 confirmed and 350 probable), the number recovered at 1,513, and the death toll 22. There are 21 active cases.
- Singapore has reported 469 new cases, bringing the total to 50,838.
- Ukraine has reported 807 new cases and 11 new deaths, bringing the total numbers to 65,656 and 1,616, respectively; a total of 36,122 patients have recovered.
- The first confirmed case of an animal infection with SARS-CoV-2 in the UK is reported, detected in a pet cat.

- Analysis from the economic forecasting group the EY Item Club suggests it will take until 2024 for the UK economy to recover from the impact of COVID-19 and the lockdown.
- The UK changes its advice on travel to Spain, advising against all non-essential travel to mainland Spain, the Balearic, and the Canary Islands.
- Transport Secretary Grant Shapps announces plans to travel home early from a family holiday in Spain due to quarantine rules.
- Travel operator Jet2 cancels all flights to mainland Spain from 28 July to 17 August.
- The number of people have tested positive for COVID-19 in the UK passes 300,000 after a further 685 positive tests bring the total number of cases to 300,111; seven deaths are also reported, the lowest daily number since 12 March, and taking the total to 45,759.
- The World Health Organisation urged all countries to make the necessary "hard choices" to avoid a new wave of lockdowns and beat the pandemic, as it announced nearly 16 million reported infection cases worldwide and over 640,000 deaths.
- The World Bank's Chief Economist for Africa, Albert Zeufack, launching a new World Bank report, urged African nations to adopt the African Continental Free Trade Area as part of coronavirus economic mitigation measures due to its potential to increase regional income by around $450 billion.
- Restaurants and nightclubs were ordered to close, and people were advised to stay at home in the Austrian town of St. Wolfgang im Salzkammergut after a recent outbreak of cases there, thought to be linked to the town's nightlife.

- Belgian Prime Minister Sophie Wilmès announced a further tightening of coronavirus restrictions in response to rising cases in the country, from July 29. Under the new restrictions, the social gathering limit will be reduced from fifteen to five people, and working from home will be "strongly encouraged" by the Belgian government. All cultural events in the worst-affected municipalities will be prohibited, with indoor venues only permitted to have a maximum audience size of 100 and outdoor venues only permitted to have 200.
- Minister-President of the German state of Bavaria Markus Söder announced that free-to-use coronavirus testing facilities will be constructed at train stations in the cities of Munich and Nuremberg, as well as at three major motorway routes near the Austria-Germany border: the border crossing at Walserberg in Austria, and near the Bavarian towns of Pocking and Kiefersfelden. German Health Minister Jens Spahn also announced that all travellers returning to Germany from countries deemed to be at a higher risk of coronavirus transmission will be required to have a mandatory test for the virus to prevent the possible importation of cases.
- Health authorities in Greece announced that the government will likely extend legislation requiring people to wear face masks in shopping centres and places of worship.
- Irish airline Ryanair reported a loss of 185 million euros in the first financial quarter of 2020 as a direct result of restrictions imposed during the coronavirus pandemic, with passenger numbers falling by as much as 99 percent.
- Spanish Foreign Affairs Minister Arancha González Laya stated that negotiations were ongoing with British authorities

to exclude the Canary Islands and Balearic Islands from the UK's 14-day quarantine measures for returning travellers, arguing that the coronavirus situation on the islands is on a similar level to in the UK.

- British Minister of State for Health and Social Care Helen Whately stated that authorities are reviewing the coronavirus situation in several countries, including France and Germany, after criticism surrounding the abrupt quarantine imposed on travellers returning from Spain by the British government.
- Indian Prime Minister Narendra Modi virtually opened three high-tech coronavirus testing facilities in Noida, Mumbai, and Kolkata, with each facility having the capacity to perform over 10,000 tests a day.
- President of Guatemala Alejandro Giammattei urged the country's population to remain vigilant as several coronavirus restrictions were lifted: shopping centres and restaurants reopened, and public transport was also permitted to resume. However, the night-time curfew and border closures remain in place.
- The majority leader of the United States Senate, Mitch McConnell, revealed further details about a coronavirus economic relief programme proposed by the Republican Party. Under the scheme, each American citizen will be entitled to $1,200; schools will receive over $100 billion in funding, more money will be injected into small businesses struggling with the financial consequences of the pandemic, $16 billion in funding was allocated to improve individual states' capacity to test for COVID-19. Over $25 billion in funding will be provided to increase the production of

personal protective equipment and potential COVID-19 vaccines in the US.

- Organisers of Major League Baseball postponed two games scheduled to be held in Miami and Philadelphia due to concerns over the coronavirus after several Miami Marlins players tested positive for COVID-19.
- CEO of Google Sundar Pichai announced that the company's employees will be encouraged to work from home until July 2021 due to surging cases worldwide.
- American biopharmaceutical company Moderna and the National Institutes of Health announced that the potential COVID-19 vaccine being developed by the two organisations and supported by the US government has moved into the late stage of human trials, involving 30,000 volunteers at nearly 90 different sites; half of the volunteers will receive small doses of the vaccine, and half will receive a placebo.
- Authorities in Lebanon re-imposed several coronavirus restrictions for a fortnight in response to a recent surge in infections in the country. Under the new restrictions, non-essential businesses including cinemas, places of worship, bars, markets, and sporting venues were ordered to close, with shops, schools, and banks only permitted to open on Tuesdays and Wednesdays. However, the country's main airport, ports, border crossings, and businesses deemed to be essential (largely medical, agricultural, industrial and governmental organisations) can remain open. All arriving international travellers will be required to enter a mandatory 48-hour quarantine to receive the results of a COVID-19 test.
- President of Kenya Uhuru Kenyatta extended the country's curfew by thirty days to reduce community transmission of coronavirus, ordered restaurants to close an hour earlier,

banned alcohol sales, and instructed bars to remain closed indefinitely. It was also announced that schools and leisure centres could potentially be converted into quarantine facilities if required.

- Nigeria's Ministry of Education announced that secondary schools will reopen from August 4 for students preparing for the West African Examination, scheduled to begin on August 17.
- The executive board of the International Monetary Fund approved $4.3 billion in financial aid to assist South African authorities in fighting the coronavirus pandemic.
- The Parliament of Zimbabwe suspended most parliamentary activities after two lawmakers tested positive for COVID-19.

29 July

- Malaysia has reported 39 new cases, bringing the total number to 8,943. Six patients have recovered, bringing the total number of recovered to 8,607. There are 212 active cases, while the death toll remains at 124.
- New Zealand has reported one new in managed isolation, bringing the total number of cases to 1,557 (1,207 confirmed and 350 probable). One person recovered, bringing the total number of recovered to 1,514. There are 21 active cases, while the death toll stands at 22.
- Singapore has reported 359 new cases, bringing the total to 51,197.
- Ukraine has reported 919 new cases and 13 new deaths, bringing the total numbers to 66,575 and 1,629, respectively; a total of 36,744 patients have recovered.

- Amid criticism that the decision to impose quarantine restrictions on people arriving from Spain is unjust, Prime Minister Boris Johnson defends the government's decision, saying further action will be taken if necessary.
- Johnson also warns that there are signs of a European second wave of the virus.
- The Andrew Lloyd Webber musical *The Phantom of the Opera* ends its 33-year run in the West End as a result of the financial impact of the COVID-19 pandemic.
- United Nations Secretary-General António Guterres launched the latest UN policy brief, COVID-19, in an Urban World, noting that cities were 'ground zero' for the pandemic and stating, "Now is the moment to adapt to the reality of this and future pandemics."
- Pakistani Prime Minister Imran Khan urged Pakistanis to continue to follow government guidelines, including social distancing and limiting contact with others over concerns that the Islamic festival of Eid al-Adha on July 31 could lead to a surge in coronavirus infections.
- American pharmaceutical company Pfizer announced that negotiations are ongoing with the European Union and several individual member states to agree on the sale of the company's potential COVID-19 vaccine.
- French Transport Minister Jean-Baptiste Djebbari stated that the government will review proposed plans to build a fourth terminal at Charles de Gaulle Airport in the capital Paris as a result of the impact of the coronavirus pandemic on the aviation industry, with the International Air Transport Association forecasting that global air traffic will not return to pre-coronavirus levels until 2024 at the earliest.

- Greek Tourism Minister Harry Theocharis announced that the ports in Athens, Corfu, Heraklion, Katakolo, Rhodes, and Volos will reopen to cruise ships from August 1.
- The Italian Senate approved legislation proposed by Prime Minister Giuseppe Conte to extend the country's state of emergency to October 15, granting the government the authority to continue to make decisions regarding the coronavirus pandemic without having to pass through parliament.
- Authorities on the Portuguese island of Madeira announced that it will be mandatory to wear a face mask in all public areas, both indoors and outdoors, from August 1 to attempt to prevent an increase in infections.
- Spanish Economy Minister Nadia Calviño announced that the government had approved 40 billion euros in credit lines to help businesses deal with the economic consequences of the coronavirus pandemic. An initial tranche of 8 billion euros was released into the Spanish economy, with 5 billion euros going to small or mid-sized businesses. The National Institute of Statistics also revealed that over one million Spanish citizens have become unemployed during the second fiscal quarter of 2020, largely from the tourism industry.
- President of the Spanish Community of Madrid Isabel Díaz Ayuso announced a tightening of coronavirus restrictions following surges in infections in several Spanish regions. From July 30, face masks will be made mandatory in all public areas of the capital city Madrid, with the only exceptions being for children under six or when exercising, and social gatherings will be limited to ten people. It was also revealed that information campaigns will target the

region's youth, to whom the spread of the virus is largely attributed.

- The Turkish government announced that schools will be permitted to reopen from August 31 as long as the daily infection rate continues to decline. To be certified as "COVID-19 secure" and be permitted to reopen, schools will be required to take several preventive measures, including regular use of hand sanitiser, temperature screening for students and staff on arrival, and ensuring that each room is well ventilated; authorities will inspect each school before it is allowed to reopen.
- Australian health authorities announced that a medical team will be sent to Papua New Guinea to assist the country in dealing with a surge in coronavirus infections. Australian Prime Minister Scott Morrison also cut short an interstate tour of Australia after reports of several large coronavirus outbreaks in nursing homes.
- Japanese automobile manufacturer Nissan reported a $2.7 billion net loss in the first fiscal quarter of 2020, warning that the company could finish the financial year with an annual net loss of $6.4 billion as a direct result of restrictions imposed to curb the spread of the coronavirus pandemic.
- Authorities in Vietnam announced that a two-week lockdown will be imposed in the city of Da Nang after a surge in domestically transmitted cases there. All public transport in and out of the city has been suspended, and tourists have been told to leave the city as soon as possible; residents must only leave their homes for important reasons, and all non-essential businesses, including beauty salons and bars, were ordered to close, with all large sporting, religious and cultural events cancelled. Authorities established several

police checkpoints to ensure that the population complies with the measures.

- Health authorities in Ecuador opened several mobile coronavirus testing centres in schools, sports stadiums, and entertainment venues in the capital Quito after the government declared a "critical situation" in the city after intensive care units reached capacity. Health Minister Juan Carlos Zevallos also announced that medical staff will be patrolling the worst-affected neighbourhoods to carry out spot tests.
- Governor of Georgia Brian Kemp withdrew his court request to prevent authorities in the state mandating the wearing of face masks in public after previously attempting to sue the mayor of Atlanta Keisha Lance Bottoms, over the decision.
- Organisers of Major League Baseball postponed all games due to be played by the Miami Marlins up to and including August 2 after seventeen of the team's players and staff tested positive for COVID-19. The MLB game between the Philadelphia Phillies and New York Yankees was also postponed after some members of the Phillies were awaiting COVID-19 test results after playing against the Marlins at the weekend.

30 July

- Malaysia has reported 13 new cases, bringing the total to 8,612. There were 10 new recoveries, bringing the total to 8,612. There are 220 active cases, while the death toll remains at 124.
- New Zealand has reported two new cases were reported in managed isolation, bringing the number of active cases to 23 and the total number of cases to 1,559 (1,209 confirmed and

350 probable). A total of 1,514 have recovered, while the death toll stands at 22.

- Singapore has reported 334 new cases, bringing the total to 51,531.
- Ukraine has reported 1,022 new cases and 21 new deaths, bringing the total numbers to 67,597 and 1,650, respectively; a total of 37,394 patients have recovered.
- Leading figures in the airline and travel industries are urging the UK government to end blanket quarantine rules impacting their sectors and instead introduce regional restrictions allowing unrestricted travel to areas of a country without significant COVID-19 outbreaks.
- The UK government announces a £500m scheme to help film and television with the costs of projects delayed or abandoned because of the COVID-19 pandemic.
- The National Trust announces plans for 1,200 redundancies in order to save £100m; the organisation estimates it has lost £200m because of the COVID-19 pandemic.
- The World Health Organization stated that the first wave of COVID-19 was continuing and that the virus was likely not impacted by seasonal changes like other respiratory diseases; it also urged significantly more respect for physical distancing measures to prevent the virus's transmission.
- The Food and Agriculture Organization issued a 'call to action highlighting the plight of hundreds of millions of smallholder family farmers in Asia-Pacific, who produce the majority of the world's food, and whose livelihoods are disproportionately suffering due to the pandemic.
- The European Commission revealed that it had paid 63 million euros to secure a limited supply of the anti-viral drug

remdesivir from the American pharmaceutical company Gilead Sciences, with orders placed to secure enough doses to treat approximately 30,000, coronavirus patients. Diplomats stated that they hope to secure more orders in the future.

- Dutch Medical Care Minister Tamara van Ark stated that the country's government will not advise residents to wear face masks in public after mixed scientific evidence received by the Health Ministry; instead, authorities will emphasise the importance of social distancing to prevent coronavirus transmission.
- The Portuguese Foreign Affairs Ministry stated that several member states of the European Union have already breached agreements aiming to ensure freedom of movement between all member countries after coronavirus lockdown restrictions were sufficiently eased to enable such a measure. Authorities cited travel restrictions to Portugal imposed by multiple countries, including Belgium, Finland, and Ireland.
- Pharmaceutical companies Sanofi and GlaxoSmithKline reached an agreement with the British government to provide up to 60 million doses of the companies' potential COVID-19 vaccine, with clinical trials scheduled to begin in September.
- Indian pharmaceutical company Hetero Drugs received approval from drug regulators to distribute its version of the anti-viral drug favipiravir, with sales scheduled to begin from August 5. This comes as a study in Mumbai found that over half of the city's slum residents had COVID-19 antibodies, implying that they have previously had the virus, raising

concerns over the accuracy of the Indian government's official data.

- Speaker of the United States House of Representatives Nancy Pelosi announced that all representatives and visitors will be required to wear face masks in the House of Representatives to prevent transmission of coronavirus after Republican Representative Louie Gohmert tested positive for COVID-19. However, members will be permitted to remove their masks when addressing the house.
- Miami-Dade County Public Schools announced that schools will not reopen physically after the summer break due to the escalating coronavirus pandemic in the US, with schools instructed to hold virtual classes from August 31.
- The Academy of Television Arts & Sciences announced that the upcoming 72nd Primetime Emmy Awards will be held virtually across the United States. It is normally held in its usual venue at Microsoft Theater in Los Angeles.
- The World Bank announced $4 billion in funding to increase the production and distribution of healthcare equipment, including personal protective equipment, ventilators, and coronavirus testing kits, to assist developing countries in fighting the pandemic.
- President of The Gambia Adama Barrow announced that he will be self-isolating for two weeks after vice-President Isatou Touray tested positive for COVID-19. Touray urged the public to wear face masks and adhere to government guidelines.
- Premier of the Australian state of Queensland Annastacia Palaszczuk announced that the state's border with Sydney will be closed from August 2 to prevent transmission of

coronavirus and that all Queensland residents returning to the state will be required to undergo a mandatory 14-day quarantine at their own expense. Australian health authorities also deployed an emergency medical team to nursing homes in the Victorian state capital of Melbourne due to a recent coronavirus outbreak there.

- Several new coronavirus restrictions came into effect in Hong Kong following consistent increases in daily infections: social gatherings of more than two people were prohibited, restaurants were forced to close all indoor areas, masks were made mandatory in all public spaces, and quarantine measures for the crew on planes and cruise ships were tightened.
- On 29 July, New Zealand Housing Minister Megan Woods announced that citizens entering the country temporarily and most non-citizens and non-residents except for family members of citizens, diplomats, or those in the country for the Christchurch mosque shootings trial would have to pay for their 14-day stay in managed isolation. However, New Zealanders intending to return home permanently will be exempt from these charges.
- Authorities in the Vietnamese capital of Hanoi ordered bars and pubs to close from midnight on July 30. They announced a ban on large social gatherings, as a result of a COVID-19 outbreak in the city of Da Nang, as well as state-owned media reporting several cases of the virus in Hanoi and Ho Chi Minh City, despite the country having previously gone three months without reporting a single domestically transmitted case.

31 July

- The Australian state of Victoria has confirmed 723 new cases and 13 deaths.
- Malaysia has reported eight new cases, bringing the total number of cases to 8,964. Five patients have recovered, bringing the total number of recovered to 8,617. The death toll remains at 124.
- New Zealand has reported one new case, bringing the number of active cases to 24 and the total number of cases to 1,560 (1,210 confirmed and 350 probable). A total of 1,514 have recovered, while the death toll remains at 22.
- Singapore has reported 278 new cases, bringing the total to 51,809.
- Ukraine has reported -high of 1,197 new daily cases and 23 new deaths, bringing the total numbers to 68,794 and 1,673, respectively; a total of 38,154 patients have recovered.
- In a bid to avoid a resurgence of COVID-19, the period for which someone testing positive for or showing signs of the virus is required to self-isolate is extended from seven to ten days.
- Prime Minister Boris Johnson warns the UK is "not out of the woods" as he warns of the danger of a resurgence.
- Restrictions are placed on Greater Manchester and parts of East Lancashire and Yorkshire, prohibiting separate households from meeting indoors following an "increasing rate of transmission" in those areas caused by people failing to adhere to social distancing rules. The restrictions take effect from midnight.
- Luxembourg is taken off the UK quarantine exemption list following a rise in COVID-19 cases.

- Office for National Statistics figures indicates England had the highest number of excess deaths in Europe between the end of February and mid-June and had the second-highest peak of deaths behind Spain.
- The Together campaign, which includes the NHS, charities, media groups, and employers, launches a consultation on how to avoid community divisions in the months ahead. The organisation has noted that the sense of community spirit fostered during lockdown is beginning to fragment.
- Cinema chain Vue announces plans to reopen some of its venues from 7 August.
- The Office for Statistics Regulation criticises First Minister of Scotland Nicola Sturgeon for comments she made in which she claimed COVID-19 rates were five times higher in England than in Scotland.
- Northern Ireland's contact tracing app StopCOVID NI was launched.
- Jet2 tells customers in the Balearic and Canary Islands to end their holidays early.
- Tui announces the closure of 166 of its high street outlets in the UK and Ireland, affecting 900 jobs.
- United Nations Secretary-General António Guterres released his latest policy brief on the coronavirus crisis (The Impact of COVID-19 on South-East Asia), which examines impacts on the 11 countries in Southeast Asia and makes recommendations for a path to sustainable, inclusive recovery that prioritises gender equality.
- The World Food Programme urgently sought international support "to prevent millions of Zimbabweans plunging

deeper into hunger" due to the COVID-19 pandemic aggravating an already severe hunger crisis in Zimbabwe.

- The Director-General of the World Health Organization warned that, while older people were among those at highest risk of COVID-19, younger generations are “not invincible.”
- The World Rugby Council approved the dates for the final rounds of the Six Nations Championship, played between England, France, Ireland, Italy, Northern Ireland, and Scotland, now scheduled to be held on October 24 and 31.
- The mayors of several French cities announced a tightening of coronavirus restrictions to prevent further transmission of the virus. In the cities of Saint-Malo and Bayonne, masks were made mandatory throughout the city with the only exceptions being for children under 11; authorities in Orleans announced that masks will be mandatory at the city's markets and in the evening along the River Loire; the resort town of Biarritz announced that masks will be compulsory in the city centre and that access to beaches will be restricted at night to prevent large gatherings.
- The Norwegian Foreign Affairs Ministry removed Belgium from a list of safe countries to travel to due to rising coronavirus cases in the country, therefore requiring all travellers returning to Norway from August 1 to enter a mandatory 10-day quarantine.
- Polish Prime Minister Mateusz Morawiecki stated that his government may re-impose quarantine measures on travellers returning to the country from several European Union member states, including France and Spain, following recent infection surges.

- British Health Secretary Matt Hancock announced that coronavirus restrictions will be tightened in Greater Manchester and parts of West Yorkshire and eastern Lancashire due to high levels of transmission. Under the new restrictions, people from different households will not be able to meet in homes or gardens and will not be allowed to mix in restaurants and pubs. The same restrictions were also imposed on the city of Leicester, in lockdown since June 30. However, restaurants, pubs, and other leisure facilities will be permitted to reopen in the city from July 31.
- Brazilian Science and Technology Minister Marcos Pontes announced that he will be working from home and self-isolating after testing positive for COVID-19, becoming the fifth minister of Jair Bolsonaro's government.
- Paraguay's Health Minister Julio Mazzoleni announced that a planned lockdown in the country's second-largest city of Ciudad del Este will be eased following violent protests. It was revealed that some non-essential businesses will be allowed to operate during the day; however, bars and gyms must still close, with all large social gatherings strictly prohibited.
- Mayor of the District of Columbia Muriel Bowser announced that schools in Washington, D.C. will not reopen as planned after the summer break due to the escalating coronavirus situation in the US and concerns from parents and teachers over the safety of reopening schools, with schools expected to organise virtual learning for students.
- Governor of Wisconsin Tony Evers declared a public health emergency and announced that face masks will be mandatory in all indoor areas due to surging coronavirus cases in the state.

- The internationally recognised Libyan government announced that a full lockdown of its territory will be imposed from August 4 following a surge in coronavirus infections and last for a minimum of five days, with people only allowed to leave their homes for strictly essential reasons.
- In the Saudi Arabian holy city of Mecca, a limited number of Islamic pilgrims participated in prayers on Mount Ararat on the peak day of the Hajj pilgrimage to enable coronavirus measures. All pilgrims were required to undergo mandatory COVID-19 tests and enter a period of self-isolation prior to the pilgrimage and must travel in groups of no more than twenty, with strict social distancing measures in place throughout.
- The Nepalese government reopened hotels, restaurants, and casinos to reduce the economic consequences of the coronavirus pandemic; permits for climbing several mountains in the Himalayas, including Mount Everest, were also issued for the first time in over four months.
- Premier of the Australian state of Victoria, Daniel Andrews, announced that face masks will be mandatory in all indoor and outdoor spaces from August 2 and that residents of the local government areas of Colac Otway, Golden Plains, Greater Geelong, Moorabool, Queenscliffe and Surf Coast will not be permitted to visit other households or have visitors in their homes in an attempt to limit the spread of coronavirus; Andrews did not rule out imposing tougher restrictions if the situation in Victoria does not improve.
- Authorities in the Chinese city of Ürümqi announced a tightening of travel restrictions following recent coronavirus outbreaks in the city. Under the new restrictions, non-residents planning on leaving the city must test negative for

COVID-19 before being permitted to leave if they have stayed there for more than two weeks in an attempt to contain the outbreak.

- Authorities in Hong Kong reversed previous legislation prohibiting restaurants from offering indoor dining due to public disapproval.
- Health officials in the Vietnamese capital of Hanoi revealed plans to perform COVID-19 tests on over 20,000 tourists who have returned from the city of Da Nang following an outbreak of domestically transmitted cases there, with residents instructed to contact their local authorities to receive a testing kit.
- In Australia, Victoria has reported 627 new cases and eight more deaths. New South Wales has reported 21 new cases, while Queensland has reported on a new case.
- Malaysia has reported 12 new cases, bringing the number of active cases to 2017 and the total number of cases to 8,976. 27 have recovered, bringing the total number to 8,644. One death was reported, bringing the death toll to 125.
- New Zealand has reported four new recoveries reported, bringing the total number of recovered to 1,518 and the number of active cases to 20. The total number of cases remains 1,560 (1,210 confirmed and 350 probable), while the death toll remains 22.
- Singapore has reported 396 new cases, bringing the total to 52,205.
- Ukraine has reported 1,090 new cases and 20 new deaths, bringing the total numbers to 69,884 and 1,693, respectively; a total of 38,752 patients have recovered.

- Prime Minister Boris Johnson postpones some lockdown easing measures scheduled to begin in England on 1 August for two weeks amid concerns about rising COVID-19 cases. Bowling alleys and casinos will remain closed until 15 August, while wedding receptions of up to 30 people are also moved back to that date. Trials of spectator sporting events are also paused. From 8 August, wearing face coverings in more indoor settings, such as cinemas and places of worship, will become mandatory.
- The ONS household survey indicates that COVID-19 cases in England are rising again, increasing from 2,800 to 4,200 daily cases in the week of 20–26 July.
- The delayed 2020 British Academy Television Awards are held as a virtual ceremony.
- Northern Ireland pauses its shielding programme.
- European pharmaceutical companies GlaxoSmithKline and Sanofi revealed that they are in advanced discussions with leaders of the European Union to provide up to 300 million doses of potential COVID-19 vaccines.
- The French National Institute of Statistics reported a record 13.8 percent decrease in the country's GDP in the second quarter of 2020, directly linked to the closure of non-essential businesses during the coronavirus pandemic.
- The German Foreign Office issued a travel warning against all non-essential travel to the Spanish autonomous communities of Aragon, Catalonia, and Navarre following surges in coronavirus infections there. All returning travellers required to receive either a COVID-19 test or enter quarantine for two weeks.

- Greek authorities announced an extension of the country's mask-wearing requirements, with face masks now mandatory in all indoor areas and outdoor areas where social distancing cannot be maintained.
- The Italian National Institute of Statistics reported that the country's GDP decreased by 12.4 percent in the second quarter of 2020 as a direct result of restrictions imposed to control the spread of coronavirus.
- Norwegian cruise Ship Company Hurtigruten instructed 160 crew and around 200 passengers who had travelled on board the Roald Amundsen to self-isolate after three crew members tested positive for COVID-19.
- Scottish First Minister Nicola Sturgeon advised the public against all non-essential travel to some northern parts of England, including the entire county of Greater Manchester, after new lockdown restrictions were imposed there following rises in rates of infection.
- British Prime Minister Boris Johnson postponed the next stage of easing coronavirus restrictions in England after rising rates of infection in several northern counties, with casinos, bowling alleys, and facial beauty salons remaining closed; it was also announced that face coverings will be mandatory in all cinemas, museums, and places of worship from August 8. England's Chief Medical Officer Chris Whitty stated that the country has "probably reached the limit of what we can do."
- Officials in the Chinese city of Ürümqi announced a further tightening of travel restrictions, with anybody arriving from areas deemed to have higher levels of coronavirus transmission required to undergo a mandatory 14-day

quarantine, with arrivals from areas with lower transmission rates required to provide evidence that they are in "good health."

- The Indonesian island of Bali reopened to domestic tourists, although international tourism cannot resume until September 11.
- President of the Philippines Rodrigo Duterte extended several coronavirus restrictions in the capital city of Manila to the middle of August due to rises in infection rates. The capital and surrounding areas were placed into a 'general community quarantine' enabling authorities to restrict the movements of the elderly and children and the operation of non-essential businesses, including gyms and restaurants. Duterte also stated that any COVID-19 vaccines available by the end of the year will be free to receive, with the poor and middle-class populations prioritised receiving them. The Philippines will receive priority from the Chinese government for vaccine distribution.
- Authorities in Vietnam recorded the country's first two coronavirus-related deaths in the city of Da Nang, raising concerns both nationally and internationally of a possible escalation of the pandemic in the country, which had gone almost three months without a domestically transmitted case before a recent outbreak. The island nation of Fiji also recorded its first coronavirus death.
- Indian automotive manufacturing company Tata Motors reported a net loss of 84 billion rupees during the second quarter of 2020 as a result of declining sales in Europe and China exacerbated by the coronavirus pandemic.
- Alicia Bárcena, head of the UN regional body for Latin America and the Caribbean (ECLAC), while noting that the

economic crisis caused by the COVID-19 pandemic was "pushing millions more into poverty," affirmed that the public health crisis had to be addressed in order to address the economic crisis.

- President of Argentina Alberto Fernández announced that further easing of coronavirus lockdown restrictions in the country would be postponed to at least August 16 due to increasing numbers of cases and concerns of healthcare facilities becoming overwhelmed.
- The US Government announced that it will pay over $2 billion to the European pharmaceutical companies GlaxoSmithKline and Sanofi to secure potential COVID-19 vaccines for 50 million Americans. The deal amounts to a total of 100 million doses, two for each patient, with the possibility of purchasing a further 500 million at a later stage, pending the results of clinical trials at the end of the year.
- Authorities in Botswana's capital city of Gaborone reimposed a coronavirus lockdown for two weeks following a surge in infections. Under the new restrictions, people are only permitted to leave their homes for essential reasons, with all social gatherings strictly prohibited; non-essential businesses, including restaurants, gyms, and hotels, were also ordered to close.
- Namibian President Hage Geingob announced that all nursery and primary schools in the country, as well as the first two years of high schools, will be closed for four weeks from August 4 to slow the spread of coronavirus, with the social gathering limit decreased from 250 to 100; restaurants and pubs will also be prohibited from selling alcohol. However, an easing of restrictions for international travellers was also announced, with arriving travellers not required to

undergo a 14-day quarantine if they present evidence of a negative COVID-19 test result taken at most three days before travel.

Pandemic Chronology August 2020

1 August

- Australia has reported 3 new deaths (two in Victoria and one in New South Wales), bringing the death toll to 201. The state of Victoria has reported 397 new cases.
- The Canadian province of Ontario has reported 124 new cases.
- Malaysia has reported 9 new cases, bringing the total number of cases to 8,985. There are 213 active cases, with two in intensive care and one of these on ventilator support. Three people have recovered, bringing the total number of recovered to 8,647. The death toll remains at 125.
- Mexico has reported a total of 46,688 deaths and 424,637 infections, giving the country the third-highest death rate from COVID-19.
- New Zealand has reported 2 new cases, bringing the number of active cases to 22 and the total number to 1,562 (1,212 confirmed and 350 probable). The number of recovered remains at 1,518, while the death toll remains at 22.
- Singapore has reported 307 new cases, bringing the total to 52,512.
- Ukraine has reported 1,172 new cases and 16 new deaths, bringing the total numbers to 71,056 and 1,709, respectively; a total of 39,308 patients have recovered.
- The shielding programme is paused for England and Scotland but will continue for the areas where extra precautions have been introduced.

- Changes to the furlough scheme come into effect, with firms who have furloughed workers required to contribute to the Coronavirus Job Retention Scheme. They must pay National Insurance and pension contributions until the scheme ends in October.
- The WHO Emergency Committee expressed "appreciation for WHO and partners' COVID-19 pandemic response efforts", while noting that there was no end in sight to a crisis that had so far infected over 17 million people and resulted in over 650,000 deaths, stressing that the impact would last for decades.
- Health officials in the Costa Rican capital of San José dispatched a mobile laboratory team to the Costa Rica-Nicaragua border to provide free COVID-19 tests to migrants stranded at the border after the Nicaraguan government announced that anybody unable to provide evidence of a negative result will be prohibited from entering the country.
- Governor of Puerto Rico Wanda Vázquez Garced extended restrictions imposed to control the spread of the coronavirus pandemic, with cinemas, bars and gyms remaining closed until at least August 15, with beaches closed to people not exercising every day except Sundays. Puerto Rico's night-time curfew was also retained with no large social gatherings permitted; authorities also stated that anybody refusing to wear a face mask in a public space could face prosecution.
- American technology company Google stated that twenty US states and territories are experimenting with contact tracing technology developed by the company, with sixteen countries already using the Exposure Notification app developed jointly by Google and Apple Inc.

- French authorities began testing travellers arriving from countries deemed to be at higher risk of coronavirus transmission at sixteen of the country's main international transport hubs after Prime Minister Jean Castex announced the measure in July, with anybody testing positive required to enter a mandatory two-week quarantine; travellers who present evidence of a negative COVID-19 test result received less than three days before travel are exempt.
- International flights to and from Russia resumed at Sheremetyevo International Airport in Moscow, and cinemas reopened at a reduced capacity across the country as part of a further easing of coronavirus restrictions; customers at cinemas were required to maintain a strict social distance and have their temperatures checked on arrival.
- Russian Health Minister Mikhail Murashko revealed governmental plans to carry out a mass vaccination campaign against COVID-19 in October, with healthcare and educational personnel announced to be the first to receive a vaccine.
- In the United Kingdom, shielding of people in vulnerable categories in England, Scotland and Northern Ireland ended, enabling those previously shielding to return to work; they will no longer be entitled to receive food parcels and medication deliveries from the government. British Prime Minister Boris Johnson also announced an easing of coronavirus restrictions scheduled to take place over the weekend would be delayed to at least August 15 following rises in infection rates in several areas of the country, with casinos, bowling alleys, facial beauty salons and indoor entertainment remaining closed.

- The Kuwaiti Directorate General of Civil Aviation banned commercial flights to over thirty countries authorities deem to have unsafe levels of coronavirus transmission. Countries to which flights were suspended include Brazil, China, Egypt, India and Spain.
- Kenya's national airline Kenya Airways resumed international flights after they were suspended in March due to the coronavirus pandemic.
- A decision by the Malaysian Government requiring people to wear face masks in public spaces and public transportation comes into effect. Under the Prevention and Control of Infectious Diseases Act, violators face a fine of up to RM1,000 (S$324).
- The Singaporean Immigration and Checkpoints Authority requires Malaysian citizens and permanent residents with Singapore work passes to serve a stay-home notice for at least seven days and undergo a COVID-19 swab test.
- French authorities began testing travellers arriving from countries deemed to be at higher risk of coronavirus transmission at sixteen of the country's main international transport hubs after Prime Minister Jean Castex announced the measure in July, with anybody testing positive required to enter a mandatory two week quarantine; travellers who present evidence of a negative COVID-19 test result received less than three days before travel are exempt.
- International flights to and from Russia resumed at Sheremetyevo International Airport in Moscow, and cinemas reopened at a reduced capacity across the country as part of a further easing of coronavirus restrictions; customers at

cinemas were required to maintain a strict social distance and have their temperatures checked on arrival.

- Russian Health Minister Mikhail Murashko revealed governmental plans to carry out a mass vaccination campaign against COVID-19 in October, with healthcare and educational personnel announced to be the first to receive a vaccine.
- In the United Kingdom, shielding of people in vulnerable categories in England, Scotland and Northern Ireland ended, enabling those previously shielding to return to work; they will no longer be entitled to receive food parcels and medication deliveries from the government. British Prime Minister Boris Johnson also announced an easing of coronavirus restrictions scheduled to take place over the weekend would be delayed to at least August 15 following rises in infection rates in several areas of the country, with casinos, bowling alleys, facial beauty salons and indoor entertainment remaining closed.
- Governor of Okinawa Prefecture in Japan, Denny Tamaki, declared a state of emergency in all of Okinawa following surges in daily coronavirus infections and authorities warning that healthcare facilities could potentially be overwhelmed. Residents were urged to avoid non-essential travel for two weeks, although the measures are not enforceable by law.
- South Korean authorities arrested Lee Man-hee, the leader of the Shincheonji Church of Jesus, on charges of obstructing the government's efforts to contain the COVID-19 pandemic in February and March 2020.
- Authorities in the Vietnamese city of Da Nang revealed plans to provide COVID-19 tests for all of the city's 1.1 million residents after a recent outbreak of domestically transmitted

infections there, with the testing capacity scheduled to be increased to up to 10,000 a day.

2 August

- The Australian state of Victoria has reported 671 new cases and 7 deaths within the last 24 hours.
- The Canadian province Of Ontario has reported 116 new cases.
- Malaysia has reported 14 new cases, bringing the total number to 8,999. 17 people recovered, bringing the total number of recoveries to 8,664. The death toll stands at 125.
- New Zealand has reported 3 new cases, bringing the number of active cases to 25 and the total number to 1,565 (1,215 confirmed and 350 probable). The number of recovered remains at 1,518, and the death toll stands at 22.
- Singapore has reported 313 new cases, bringing the total to 52,825.
- Ukraine has reported 1,112 new cases and 16 new deaths, bringing the total numbers to 72,168 and 1,725, respectively; a total of 39,543 patients have recovered.
- A major incident is declared in Greater Manchester after rises in coronavirus infection rates.
- The Cypriot Health Ministry announced that all travellers arriving into the country from Greece from August 5 would be required to receive a mandatory COVID-19 test if they cannot produce evidence of a negative test result received less than three days before arrival, following a surge in infections in Greece.
- French authorities stated that they would request for European Union leaders to impose financial sanctions on

any member state undermining basic human rights under the union's coronavirus pandemic recovery fund.

- In the United Kingdom, the Greater Manchester Combined Authority declared a major incident throughout the county after the British government announced that coronavirus restrictions would be tightened in the area. Authorities later stated that the major incident was declared to enable key organisations to access resources to prevent further transmission of the virus.
- Indian Home Affairs Minister Amit Shah tested positive for COVID-19 and subsequently urged everybody who had been in close contact with him to self-isolate at home.
- In Australia, Premier of Victoria Daniel Andrews announced that the state of Victoria will enter into a state of emergency from 6 pm Sunday local time after 671 new cases were reported that day. Melbourne will enter into "stage four" lockdown restrictions on travel and businesses, with only one person per household allowed out to go shopping each day, with schools asked to hold lessons remotely. Regional areas will move into "stage three restrictions", with cafes and restaurants being allowed to provide takeaway services.
- China's National Health Commission dispatched a team of officials to Hong Kong, experiencing a third wave of infections, to conduct mass COVID-19 testing.
- President of the Philippines, Rodrigo Duterte, announced that the coronavirus lockdown in the Greater Manila Area will be significantly tightened from August 4 following surging coronavirus infections. The lockdown in the area was upgraded to a "Modified Enhanced Community Quarantine" until at least August 18; under the new restrictions, residents will be forced to only travel for essential reasons, with all

public transport being suspended, and hairdressers, beauty salons, and gyms will all close, although shopping centres and restaurants can remain open at reduced capacities.

- White House Chief of Staff Mark Meadows stated that he was not optimistic that American politicians will reach an agreement in the near future on further legislation aimed at relieving economic pressure on families and businesses affected by the pandemic.
- The Cypriot Health Ministry announced that all travellers arriving into the country from Greece from August 5 will be required to receive a mandatory COVID-19 test if they cannot produce evidence of a negative test result received less than three days before arrival, following a surge in infections in Greece.
- French authorities stated that they would request for European Union leaders to impose financial sanctions on any member state undermining basic human rights under the union's coronavirus pandemic recovery fund.
- In the United Kingdom, the Greater Manchester Combined Authority declared a major incident throughout the county after the British government announced that coronavirus restrictions will be tightened in the area. Authorities later stated that the major incident was declared to enable key organisations to access resources to prevent further transmission of the virus.
- Iraq's Civil Aviation Authority suspended all flights between Iraq and Turkey following a surge in coronavirus infections in Turkey.

3 August

- The Australian state of Victoria has reported 429 new cases and 13 deaths, bringing the total number of active cases in Victoria to 6,489.
- The Canadian Province of Ontario has reported 88 new cases.
- Malaysia has reported 2 new cases, bringing the total number to 9,001. Four patients were discharged, bringing the number of recovered to 8,670. There are 208 active cases, while the death toll stands at 125.
- New Zealand has reported 2 new cases in managed isolation, bringing the total number of active cases to 27 and the total number to 1,567 (1,217 confirmed and 350 probable). The number of recovered remains at 1,518, and the death toll stands at 22.
- Singapore has reported 226 new cases, bringing the total to 53,051.
- Ukraine has reported 990 new cases and 13 new deaths, bringing the total numbers to 73,158 and 1,738, respectively; a total of 39,876 patients have recovered.
- The month-long "Eat Out to Help Out" scheme begins, offering a 50% discount on meals at indoor venues, three days per week, with the remainder of the cost picked up by the government.
- Restaurants, pubs and hairdressers in Leicester are allowed to reopen as lockdown restrictions are eased in the city.
- The World Health Organization's Emergency Committee on COVID-19 met to review the current coronavirus pandemic at what Director-General Tedros Adhanom Ghebreyesus

called “a sobering moment” due to the pandemic's massive direct and ripple effects, with a warning of "no silver bullet".

- UNICEF warned that storms and coronavirus posed a ‘double threat’ for children in Central America and the Caribbean.
- The World Health Organization’s Emergency Committee on COVID-19 met to review the current coronavirus pandemic at what Director-General Tedros Adhanom Ghebreyesus called “a sobering moment” due to the pandemic's massive direct and ripple effects, with a warning of "no silver bullet".
- UNICEF warned that storms and coronavirus posed a ‘double threat’ for children in Central America and the Caribbean.
- In The Gambia, Finance Minister Mambury Njie, Energy Minister Fafa Sanyang, and Agriculture Minister Amie Fabureh all tested positive for COVID-19 and will subsequently self-isolate and work from home, taking the total number of cabinet ministers infected with the virus to five.
- South Africa's anti-corruption organisation announced that it was investigating irregularities in several aspects of the government's handling of the coronavirus pandemic, amid concerns that senior officials have gained access to millions of rand of financial aid.
- Health authorities in the French cities of Lille and Nice announced that face masks will be mandatory in all outdoor public spaces, in addition to all indoor areas, to attempt to lower the rate of coronavirus transmission; police in Lille stated that anybody caught breaking the regulations on face masks will receive a fine of 135 euros. French Prime Minister

Jean Castex also urged the public to remain vigilant, stating that "the virus is not on holiday and neither are we".

- Schools reopened in the German state of Mecklenburg-Vorpommern with no requirement for students to wear face masks, despite Education Minister Anja Karliczek advocating such a measure.
- Authorities in Greece announced that face masks will be mandatory on outdoor areas on board ships until August 18, following a surge in infections in the country.
- Polish Health Minister Łukasz Szumowski stated that law enforcement officers will be performing checks on shops to ensure they are complying with the government's COVID-19 restrictions.
- Norwegian Health Minister Bent Høie announced that cruise ships carrying more than 100 passengers will be prohibited from disembarking at Norwegian ports for two weeks, after more than 40 passengers and crew tested positive on board the MS Roald Amundsen. The new restrictions will not apply to scheduled domestic and international ferry companies. The operator of the MS Roald Amundsen Hurtigruten announced that all of the company's cruises will be suspended until further notice.
- The Shri Ram Janmabhoomi Teerth Kshetra, the trust established to manage the construction of the Ram Mandir temple in Ayodhya, stated that preparations were still going ahead for the Indian Prime Minister Narendra Modi's visit to the site on August 5, despite the escalating coronavirus situation in the country.
- Indian biopharmaceutical company Wockhardt announced that it had reached an agreement with the British

government to supply millions of doses of several different COVID-19 vaccines; the company also revealed that it had reserved the final stage of manufacturing of the vaccines as part of the agreement. Manufacturing will be carried out at the site of CP Pharmaceuticals, a subsidiary company of Wockhardt, in Wrexham.

- In The Gambia, Finance Minister Mambury Njie, Energy Minister Fafa Sanyang, and Agriculture Minister Amie Fabureh all tested positive for COVID-19 and will subsequently self-isolate and work from home, taking the total number of cabinet ministers infected with the virus to five.
- South Africa's anti-corruption organisation announced that it was investigating irregularities in several aspects of the government's handling of the coronavirus pandemic, amid concerns that senior officials have gained access to millions of rand of financial aid.
- On 3 August, Victorian Premier Daniel Andrews announced that supermarkets, grocery stores, pharmacies, petrol stations, banks, news agencies, post offices, and other businesses involved in the state's pandemic response would be allowed to remain open, although the retail sector and some manufacturing and administrative companies will be closed from midnight on 5 August. The meat processing and construction industries would be allowed to operate with reduced personnel.
- The Singaporean Immigration and Checkpoints Authority announced that all travellers arriving or returning to the country from August 11 will be required to wear an electronic monitoring device to ensure that they comply with coronavirus regulations, with attempts to leave the

mandatory two weeks quarantine or alter the device's settings alerting authorities.

- Chief of Staff in the Brazilian Presidency Walter Souza Braga Netto tested positive for COVID-19 and will subsequently self-isolate and work from home, making him the seventh government minister to contract coronavirus.
- Authorities in Honduras extended the country's coronavirus curfew by a further week, now scheduled to end on August 9, due to rising rates of infection both domestically and internationally.
- In the United States, staff in over thirty school districts organised protests against the American government's plans to fully reopen schools at the end of the summer break due to surging coronavirus cases in the country; they urged the government to reconsider the plans and allow lessons to be held virtually until there is substantial scientific evidence supporting the physical reopening of schools, with several safety measures implemented such as the wearing of face masks and smaller class sizes.
- The Australian state of Victoria has reported 439 new cases and 11 deaths.
- The Canadian province of Ontario has reported 91 new cases.
- Malaysia has reported 1 new case, bringing the total number to 9,002. There are 193 active cases and a total of 8,684 recoveries.
- New Zealand has reported five new recoveries, bringing the total number of recovered to 1,523. There are 22 active cases, with the total number of cases remaining 1,567 (1,217 confirmed and 350 probable) and the death toll at 22.

- Singapore has reported 295 new cases, bringing the total to 53,346.
- Ukraine has reported 1,061 new cases and 26 new deaths, bringing the total numbers to 74,219 and 1,764, respectively; a total of 40,613 patients have recovered.

4 August

- Scientists warn that test and trace provisions are inadequate to prevent a second wave of COVID-19 once schools reopen in September.
- Secretary-General António Guterres issued recommendations to get children back in the classroom in a new UNESCO policy brief, Education During COVID-19 And Beyond: "The Future Of Education Is Here", launched alongside a new global campaign called Save our Future, as the UN estimates 1 billion children were affected by school closures in July.
- The UN launched a COVID-19 Response Plan for the Philippines to provide "critical health interventions and multi-sectoral humanitarian assistance" to those in epidemic hotspots in its largest country response since 2013, the UN response to Typhoon Haiyan/Yolanda.
- The German government lifted warnings advising against travel to the Turkish coastal regions of Antalya, Aydın, İzmir, and Muğla.
- Irish Taoiseach Micheál Martin delayed moving the country into the fourth phase of reopening after the coronavirus pandemic by three weeks, meaning that bars, pubs and casinos will remain closed, and restrictions on the size of social gatherings will not change as planned.

- The Turkish Interior Ministry announced that new inspection and enforcement rules will come into immediate effect in over 80 of the country's provinces to ensure that the public and businesses are complying with coronavirus restrictions after a recent surge in infections. Authorities also stated that tougher restrictions may be implemented in the capital Ankara to slow the spread of the virus.
- The mayor of Kanifing District in The Gambia, Talib Bensouda, tested positive for COVID-19 and was admitted to hospital for treatment, becoming the sixth senior politician in the country to test positive.
- Nigerian private airline Air Peace announced that salaries have been cut and that around 70 pilots have been made redundant due to the impact of the COVID-19 pandemic on aviation.
- Vice-President of Zimbabwe Constantino Chiwenga was announced as the country's new Health Minister, following the dismissal of previous minister Obadiah Moyo over several corruption allegations relating to the government's handling of the coronavirus pandemic.
- Secretary-General of the Brazilian Presidency Jorge de Oliveira Francisco tested positive for COVID-19 and will subsequently work from home, becoming the eighth cabinet minister to test positive.
- The United States Government announced that late-stage clinical trials have begun of a potential antibody treatment and several experimental therapeutics for treating moderately-affected COVID-19 patients, developed jointly by Canadian biotechnology company AbCellera and American firm Eli Lilly and Company.

- Bulgarian health authorities announced that fans will be permitted to return to sports stadiums as long as they take up no more than fifty per cent of the venue's capacity when the First Professional Football League resumes on August 7.
- French President Emmanuel Macron announced that each care home worker in France will be entitled to receive a bonus of 500 euros as a show of gratitude for their role in fighting the coronavirus pandemic; the overall package will be worth 160 billion euros, half of which will be funded by the French national government and half by local governments.
- The German government lifted warnings advising against travel to the Turkish coastal regions of Antalya, Aydın, İzmir, and Muğla.
- Irish Taoiseach Micheál Martin delayed moving the country into the fourth phase of reopening after the coronavirus pandemic by three weeks, meaning that bars, pubs and casinos will remain closed, and restrictions on the size of social gatherings will not change as planned.
- Indian health authorities announced that phase two clinical trials have begun of two different potential COVID-19 vaccines, developed by biotechnology company Bharat Biotech and pharmaceutical company Cadila Healthcare respectively.
- Victorian Premier Daniel Andrews announced that those who are self-isolating will only be allowed to exercise within their own properties. Australian Defence Force and Victorian Department of Health and Human Services officers would also be visiting homes to ensure that people are complying with self-isolation orders, with anyone breaching the orders possibly fined up to 20,000 Australian dollars.

- Australian authorities extended the closure of the Uluṟu-Kata Tjuṯa National Park due to concerns from the indigenous population that visitors could potentially spread the coronavirus to the area, with the indigenous community believed to be at a considerably higher risk of developing severe symptoms.
- Stay-at-home orders were issued on the Philippine island of Luzon, including in the capital city of Manila, following a surge in coronavirus infections, effectively placing thirty million people back into lockdown. The order will be in effect for two weeks, with residents only permitted to leave their homes for strictly essential reasons; restaurants were instructed to close all indoor dining areas, and all public transport on the island was suspended.
- The Taiwan Centers for Disease Control provisionally approved the use of dexamethasone to treat COVID-19 patients due to global shortages of the remdesivir drug.
- Indian health authorities announced that phase two clinical trials have begun of two different potential COVID-19 vaccines, developed by biotechnology company Bharat Biotech and pharmaceutical company Cadila Healthcare respectively.
- The mayor of Kanifing District in The Gambia, Talib Bensouda, tested positive for COVID-19 and was admitted to hospital for treatment, becoming the sixth senior politician in the country to test positive.
- Nigerian private airline Air Peace announced that salaries have been cut and that around 70 pilots have been made redundant due to the impact of the COVID-19 pandemic on aviation.

- Vice-President of Zimbabwe Constantino Chiwenga was announced as the country's new Health Minister, following the dismissal of previous minister Obadiah Moyo over several corruption allegations relating to the government's handling of the coronavirus pandemic.

5 August

- The Australian state of Victoria has reported 725 new cases, bringing the total to 13,035. 15 new deaths were reported, bringing the state's death toll to 162.
- The Canadian province of Ontario has reported 86 new cases.
- Malaysia has reported 21 new cases, bringing the total number to 9,023. 18 have recovered, bringing the total number of recovered to 8,702.
- New Zealand has 2 new cases, bringing the number of active cases to 24 and the total number to 1,569 (1,219 confirmed and 350 probable). The number of recovered and death remains 1,523 and 22 respectively.
- Singapore has reported 908 new cases, bringing the total to 54,254.
- Ukraine has reported record-high 1,271 new daily cases as well as 24 new deaths, bringing the total numbers to 75,490 and 1,788 respectively; a total of 41,527 patients have recovered.
- A report by the Home Affairs committee concludes that the spread of COVID-19 could have been slowed by an earlier implementation of quarantine restrictions on people arriving in the UK.

- Bank of Ireland announces plans for 1,400 job losses collectively from its UK and Ireland operations.
- The World Health Organization reported that a new "surge team" of leading UN health experts was travelling to South Africa to help with the COVID-19 response there, as the country was now among the top five of the world's most affected countries.
- The German Foreign Office advised against all non-essential travel to the Belgian province of Antwerp and declared the city of Antwerp to be a high-risk area, with all travellers returning to Germany required to enter a 14-day quarantine.
- Health authorities in the Dutch capital of Amsterdam announced that it will be mandatory to wear a face mask in several popular outdoor areas of the city, including the De Wallen red-light district.
- Data from Statistics Sweden revealed that the country's GDP contracted by 8.6 per cent in the second quarter of 2020, the largest decrease since 1980.
- Health authorities in Switzerland added The Bahamas, Equatorial Guinea, Romania, São Tomé and Príncipe, Singapore and mainland Spain to a list of countries deemed to have unsafe levels of coronavirus transmission, therefore requiring all travellers returning to Switzerland from August 8 to enter a mandatory quarantine. Azerbaijan, Russia and the United Arab Emirates were removed from the list; authorities also added pregnant women to the vulnerable category and strongly advised them against extended close contact with people outside of their household.
- Scottish First Minister Nicola Sturgeon reimposed several lockdown restrictions in the city of Aberdeen following a rise

in infections linked to nightlife in the city. Therefore, restaurants and pubs were instructed to close with immediate effect. Authorities advised against non-essential travel, with residents prohibited from visiting other households; the measures will be reviewed on August 12 and extended if deemed necessary.

- Canadian Procurement Minister Anita Anand announced that the government had reached an agreement with American pharmaceutical companies Pfizer and Moderna to secure millions of doses of potential COVID-19 vaccines; Anand also stated that negotiations were ongoing with several other domestic and international companies to secure doses.
- In the United States, data from the ADP National Employment Report shows that only 170,000 private company employees were hired in July, a stark contrast to over 4 million hired in June, with data also suggesting that there are 13 million fewer people employed in the US than in February, attributed directly to the economic impact of the coronavirus pandemic.
- The Chicago Teachers Union announced that schools will not reopen physically after the summer break in September, with lessons conducted online to prevent coronavirus transmission.
- Mayor of New York City Bill de Blasio announced that coronavirus checkpoints will be established on major entry points to New York City to ensure that travellers arriving from states deemed to have unsafe levels of transmission stay in quarantine for two weeks, with fines of up to $10,000 for anyone caught breaching the orders.
- Gambian President Adama Barrow declared a state of emergency in the country due to a large surge in coronavirus

infections, closing the country's land, sea and air borders to everyone except diplomatic staff and essential delivery drivers. Schools and places of worship were also closed, although essential businesses were permitted to reopen. A night-time curfew was also introduced for three weeks to attempt to lower the transmission of the virus.

- Authorities in Oman announced that a ban on domestic travel between the country's provinces will be lifted on August 8 after it was initially imposed to control possible coronavirus transmission during the Islamic festival of Eid al-Adha. The country's curfew will also be shortened for a week, although all restrictions in Dhofar Governorate will be maintained.
- Gambian President Adama Barrow declared a state of emergency in the country due to a large surge in coronavirus infections, closing the country's land, sea and air borders to everyone except diplomatic staff and essential delivery drivers. Schools and places of worship were also closed, although essential businesses were permitted to reopen. A night-time curfew was also introduced for three weeks to attempt to lower the transmission of the virus.
- Premier of the Australian state of Queensland Annastacia Palaszczuk announced that the borders with New South Wales and the Australian Capital Territory will be closed from August 8 to attempt to prevent the spread of coronavirus.
- In China, human trials of a potential COVID-19 vaccine, developed jointly by German company BioNTech and Chinese company Fosun Pharmaceutical began with over seventy participants.

- Statistics Indonesia revealed that the Indonesian GDP contracted by 5.3 per cent in the second quarter of 2020, the largest decline since the 1997 Asian financial crisis.
- The German Foreign Office advised against all non-essential travel to the Belgian province of Antwerp and declared the city of Antwerp to be a high-risk area, with all travellers returning to Germany required to enter a 14-day quarantine.
- Health authorities in the Dutch capital of Amsterdam announced that it will be mandatory to wear a face mask in several popular outdoor areas of the city, including the De Wallen red-light district.
- Data from Statistics Sweden revealed that the country's GDP contracted by 8.6 per cent in the second quarter of 2020, the largest decrease since 1980.
- Health authorities in Switzerland added The Bahamas, Equatorial Guinea, Romania, São Tomé and Príncipe, Singapore and mainland Spain to a list of countries deemed to have unsafe levels of coronavirus transmission, therefore requiring all travellers returning to Switzerland from August 8 to enter a mandatory quarantine. Azerbaijan, Russia and the United Arab Emirates were removed from the list; authorities also added pregnant women to the vulnerable category and strongly advised them against extended close contact with people outside of their household.
- Scottish First Minister Nicola Sturgeon reimposed several lockdown restrictions in the city of Aberdeen following a rise in infections linked to nightlife in the city. Therefore, restaurants and pubs were instructed to close with immediate effect. Authorities advised against non-essential travel, with residents prohibited from visiting other

households; the measures will be reviewed on August 12 and extended if deemed necessary.

- The World Health Organization reported that a new "surge team" of leading UN health experts was travelling to South Africa to help with the COVID-19 response there, as the country was now among the top five of the world's most affected countries.

6 August

- The Australian state of Victoria has reported 471 new cases and 8 new deaths, bringing the death toll to 170. In addition, 107 "mystery cases" had emerged while 1,533 active cases were linked to aged care facilities.
- The Canadian province of Ontario has reported 95 new cases.
- Malaysia has reported 15 new cases, bringing the total number to 9,038. 11 have recovered, bringing the total number of recovered to 8,713. There are 200 active cases, while the death toll remains at 125.
- New Zealand has reported no new cases, with the total number of cases remaining 1,569 (1,219 confirmed and 350 probable cases). One new recovery was reported, bringing the total number to 1,524. There are 23 active cases, while the death toll remains 22.
- Singapore has reported 301 new cases, bringing the total to 54,555.
- Ukraine has reported a record-high 1,318 new daily cases and repeated the previously set record of 31 new daily deaths, bringing the total numbers to 76,808 and 1,819, respectively; a total of 42,524 patients have recovered.

- Quarantine restrictions are placed on travellers arriving into the UK from Belgium, the Bahamas and Andorra, with the new rules coming into effect from midnight in Wales, and 4 am on 8 August in the rest of the UK.
- The Bank of England predicts that the economic impact of the COVID-19 pandemic will be less severe than previously thought, but the economy will take much longer than anticipated to recover.
- Organisers of the 2020 London Marathon, scheduled for 4 October, announced it is to be an elite athletes only event due to the COVID-19 pandemic, with the race taking place on a bio-secure course.
- Addressing the Aspen Security Forum, consisting of top-level present and former United States government officials, Tedros Adhanom Ghebreyesus, Director-General of the World Health Organization (WHO), appealed to countries to unite against the disease, stressing that there were more than 18.5 million cases of COVID-19 worldwide and 700,000 deaths.
- The UN World Food Programme (WFP) and governments announced that a flight carrying "protective masks, ventilators and other essential medical supplies for COVID-19 response" had landed in Papua New Guinea, commencing a humanitarian air service for the Pacific region.
- Danish Health Minister Magnus Heunicke announced that the limit on social gatherings will not be lifted following a recent surge in new infections across the country, on advice from the Statens Serum Institut.

- Dutch Prime Minister Mark Rutte stated that authorities were not considering imposing a second coronavirus lockdown despite rising infection rates in several parts of the country; he also urged tourists to avoid busier areas of the capital Amsterdam and for people to observe social distancing at all times.
- Norwegian authorities advised against all non-essential travel to the Czech Republic, France, Monaco and Switzerland due to rising coronavirus cases, therefore requiring all travellers returning from those countries to Norway to enter a mandatory 10-day quarantine. Health Minister Bent Høie also announced that the same measures would apply to the Swedish counties of Skåne and Kronoberg, although the counties of Dalarna, Södermanland, Uppsala and Västerbotten would be removed from the quarantine list.
- British Transport Secretary Grant Shapps announced that Andorra, the Bahamas and Belgium will be removed from the government's list of safe countries to travel to due to rising rates of infection, therefore requiring all travellers returning to the UK to self-isolate for 14 days. Shapps also announced that travellers returning from Brunei and Malaysia would no longer have to self-isolate.
- First Minister of Northern Ireland Arlene Foster delayed the reopening of pubs to an 'indicative date' of September 1 and announced that face masks will be compulsory in shops from August 10, as a result of the basic reproduction number rising above 1. Foster also confirmed that schools in Northern Ireland will fully reopen after the summer break at the start of September.

- Organisers of the 2020 London Marathon announced that the event will feature only elite runners and wheelchair racers due to public health concerns. Runners who had been scheduled to participate will be able to engage in a virtual marathon instead.
- The Australian city of Melbourne entered a six-week coronavirus lockdown to attempt to slow the rapidly increasing spread of the virus. Under the new restrictions, all non-essential businesses were closed, and residents were instructed to stay at home unless travel was strictly essential.
- Japanese automobile manufacturer Toyota reported a profit of 13.9 billion yen for the first fiscal quarter of 2020, down 98 per cent, which was attributed to the impact of the coronavirus pandemic.
- Managers at the Ok Tedi Mine in Papua New Guinea announced that the company would suspend operations for at least two weeks after a number of cases were reported amongst employees.
- The Philippine Statistics Authority revealed data that shows how the country's gross domestic product growth rate decreased by 16.5 per cent in the second quarter of 2020, the biggest contraction since records began in 1981. This officially placed the Philippine economy into recession, the first time the economy has been in recession in over thirty years.
- Pakistani Planning Minister Asad Umar announced that several coronavirus restrictions will be eased following a decrease in the number of new infections. Restaurants, cafes, theme parks, gyms, theatres, cinemas and casinos

will be permitted to reopen from August 10, and wedding venues and schools will reopen from September 15. Restrictions on public transport will also be eased, although the number of passengers able to travel will remain restricted until October.

- Danish Health Minister Magnus Heunicke announced that the limit on social gatherings will not be lifted following a recent surge in new infections across the country, on advice from the Statens Serum Institut.
- Dutch Prime Minister Mark Rutte stated that authorities were not considering imposing a second coronavirus lockdown despite rising infection rates in several parts of the country; he also urged tourists to avoid busier areas of the capital Amsterdam and for people to observe social distancing at all times.
- Norwegian authorities advised against all non-essential travel to the Czech Republic, France, Monaco and Switzerland due to rising coronavirus cases, therefore requiring all travellers returning from those countries to Norway to enter a mandatory 10-day quarantine. Health Minister Bent Høie also announced that the same measures would apply to the Swedish counties of Skåne and Kronoberg, although the counties of Dalarna, Södermanland, Uppsala and Västerbotten would be removed from the quarantine list.
- British Transport Secretary Grant Shapps announced that Andorra, the Bahamas and Belgium will be removed from the government's list of safe countries to travel to due to rising rates of infection, therefore requiring all travellers returning to the UK to self-isolate for 14 days. Shapps also

announced that travellers returning from Brunei and Malaysia would no longer have to self-isolate.

- First Minister of Northern Ireland Arlene Foster delayed the reopening of pubs to an 'indicative date' of September 1 and announced that face masks will be compulsory in shops from August 10, as a result of the basic reproduction number rising above 1. Foster also confirmed that schools in Northern Ireland will fully reopen after the summer break at the start of September.
- Organisers of the 2020 London Marathon announced that the event will feature only elite runners and wheelchair racers due to public health concerns. Runners who had been scheduled to participate will be able to engage in a virtual marathon instead.
- Nigerian Aviation Minister Hadi Sirika stated that commercial international flights to and from the country will be permitted to resume in "weeks rather than months".
- South African President Cyril Ramaphosa announced that a committee will be established to investigate alleged corruption linked to the government's handling of the coronavirus pandemic, as well as businesses supplying personal protective equipment.
- Researchers at Padjadjaran University in the Indonesian city of Bandung announced that the first human trials of a potential COVID-19 vaccine involving over 1,500 volunteers will begin on August 11, developed jointly by a Chinese biopharmaceutical company Sinovac Biotech and Indonesian vaccine manufacturer Bio Farma.
- Pakistani Planning Minister Asad Umar announced that several coronavirus restrictions will be eased following a

decrease in the number of new infections. Restaurants, cafes, theme parks, gyms, theatres, cinemas and casinos will be permitted to reopen from August 10, and wedding venues and schools will reopen from September 15. Restrictions on public transport will also be eased, although the number of passengers able to travel will remain restricted until October.

- Addressing the Aspen Security Forum, consisting of top-level present and former United States government officials, Tedros Adhanom Ghebreyesus, Director-General of the World Health Organization (WHO), appealed to countries to unite against the disease, stressing that there were more than 18.5 million cases of COVID-19 worldwide and 700,000 deaths.
- The UN World Food Programme (WFP) and governments announced that a flight carrying "protective masks, ventilators and other essential medical supplies for COVID-19 response" had landed in Papua New Guinea, commencing a humanitarian air service for the Pacific region.
- The Supreme Federal Court of Brazil ruled that President Jair Bolsonaro must impose measures to prevent the spread of coronavirus to the country's indigenous communities, widely understood to be at a higher risk of developing severe cases of COVID-19. The government was given thirty days to implement suitable measures and should include barriers to stop non-residents entering tribal lands.
- United States President Donald Trump stated that the US could potentially have a COVID-19 vaccine by November 3, the date of the 2020 presidential election.

- Governor of Ohio Mike DeWine tested positive for COVID-19 and will subsequently self-isolate and work from his home in Cedarville.
- The United States Department of State lifted the Global Level 4 Health Advisory, which advised citizens against all non-essential international travel, based on data from the Centers for Disease Control and Prevention.

7 August

- The Australian state of Victoria has reported 450 new cases, bringing the state's total to 13,867. The infected include 911 health workers.
- India has reported 2,027,000 confirmed cases, including 41,585 deaths.
- The Canadian province of Ontario has reported 88 new cases.
- Malaysia has reported 25 new cases, bringing the total number to 9,063. 15 have recovered, bringing the total number of recoveries to 8,728. The death toll remains at 125.
- New Zealand has reported no new cases, with the number of active cases remaining 23 and the total number of cases remaining 1,569 (1,219 confirmed and 350 probable cases). The number of recovered remains 1,524, and the death toll remains 22.
- Singapore has reported 242 new cases, bringing the total to 54,797. In addition, the Inter-agency Taskforce has completed testing in all foreign worker dormitories except for a few standalone blocks serving as quarantine facilities.

- Ukraine has reported a record-high 1,453 new daily cases as well as a record high 33 new daily deaths, bringing the total numbers to 78,261 and 1,852, respectively; a total of 43,055 patients have recovered.
- As the Americas remained the epicenter of the COVID-19 pandemic, and on the International Day of the World's Indigenous Peoples, the UN High Commissioner for Human Rights affirmed: "the need to ensure the world's indigenous people have control over their own communities", given the "critical threat" of COVID-19 to indigenous peoples.
- Special Rapporteurs and Independent Experts, part of the Special Procedures of the Human Rights Council, again called on countries to ease or lift sanctions to allow affected countries and communities "like Cuba, Iran, Sudan, Syria, Venezuela and Yemen" access vital supplies in the fight against the COVID-19 pandemic.
- Irish Taoiseach Micheál Martin announced that County Kildare, County Laois and County Offaly will be placed into Ireland's first regional lockdown for two weeks due to surging coronavirus cases there. Under the new restrictions, residents were advised to travel for essential reasons only and work from home where possible; restaurants and cafes were instructed to close all indoor dining areas, and social gatherings were limited to fifteen people outdoors and six people indoors. Casinos, cinemas, gyms, swimming pools, theatres and sporting venues were also instructed to close.
- Maltese Prime Minister Robert Abela ordered several coronavirus restrictions to be reimposed to control a surge in cases throughout the country, with face masks made mandatory in all public spaces, with fines of up to fifty euros if caught breaking the rules. Social gatherings will be limited

to 100 people indoors and 300 people outdoors, with access to care homes limited.

- Officials at Vnukovo International Airport in the Russian capital of Moscow introduced a COVID-19 express testing system, whereby arriving and departing travellers can pay to receive a COVID-19 test and receive the results within an hour.
- Spanish authorities placed the municipality of Aranda de Duero under new lockdown restrictions to slow the spread of coronavirus. Residents will be prevented from leaving the area, and non-residents will be barred from entering.
- Swiss authorities reached an agreement with the American biotechnology company Moderna to secure 4.5 million doses of the company's potential COVID-19 vaccine.
- British authorities imposed several lockdown restrictions on the city of Preston after a surge in the rate of infection there; under the restrictions, people from different households will not be allowed to meet indoors or in private gardens.
- As the Americas remained the epicenter of the COVID-19 pandemic, and on the International Day of the World's Indigenous Peoples, the UN High Commissioner for Human Rights affirmed: "the need to ensure the world’s indigenous people have control over their own communities", given the "critical threat" of COVID-19 to indigenous peoples.
- Special Rapporteurs and Independent Experts, part of the Special Procedures of the Human Rights Council, again called on countries to ease or lift sanctions to allow affected countries and communities "like Cuba, Iran, Sudan, Syria, Venezuela and Yemen" access vital supplies in the fight against the COVID-19 pandemic.

- The England and Wales Cricket Board announced that the tour of India by the England cricket team will be postponed to 2021 due to surging coronavirus cases in the country, with authorities reporting more than 2 million total cases so far.
- A court in the Indian city of Mumbai ruled that actors and crew over the age of 65 will be permitted to resume production of Bollywood films.
- Brazilian President Jair Bolsonaro announced that 1.9 billion real (equivalent to $356 million) will be allocated to the development of a potential COVID-19 vaccine by the University of Oxford and AstraZeneca, with Health Minister Eduardo Pazuello stating that the vaccine could be available as early as December.
- Governor of New York Andrew Cuomo announced that the state's schools will reopen fully after the summer break due to declining coronavirus cases, although some virtual lessons will still take place.
- The R number for the UK rises to between 0.8 and 1.0, up from the previous week's number of 0.8–0.9, but is believed to be above 1.0 in three parts of England – London, the South West and the North West.
- ITV confirms that the 2020 series of its reality programme *I'm a Celebrity...Get Me Out of Here!* will be relocated from its usual venue in the Australian jungle to a ruined castle in the UK.
- The England and Wales Cricket Board announced that the tour of India by the England cricket team will be postponed to 2021 due to surging coronavirus cases in the country, with authorities reporting more than 2 million total cases so far.

- A court in the Indian city of Mumbai ruled that actors and crew over the age of 65 will be permitted to resume production of Bollywood films.
- Chief Executive of Hong Kong Carrie Lam announced that all residents of Hong Kong will be able to access free COVID-19 tests if they wish, with Lam stating that the scheme will likely be in operation within two weeks.
- The South African Rugby Union announced that approval had been given for full-contact training sessions and games, and therefore organisers were aiming to restart tournaments in September.
- Kenyan President Uhuru Kenyatta stated that the country's hospitality industry was ready to receive both domestic and international travellers and thus urged Kenyans to travel in order to reduce the economic consequences of the COVID-19 pandemic.
- Irish Taoiseach Micheál Martin announced that County Kildare, County Laois and County Offaly will be placed into Ireland's first regional lockdown for two weeks due to surging coronavirus cases there. Under the new restrictions, residents were advised to travel for essential reasons only and work from home where possible; restaurants and cafes were instructed to close all indoor dining areas, and social gatherings were limited to fifteen people outdoors and six people indoors. Casinos, cinemas, gyms, swimming pools, theatres and sporting venues were also instructed to close.
- Maltese Prime Minister Robert Abela ordered several coronavirus restrictions to be reimposed to control a surge in cases throughout the country, with face masks made mandatory in all public spaces, with fines of up to fifty euros

if caught breaking the rules. Social gatherings will be limited to 100 people indoors and 300 people outdoors, with access to care homes limited.

- Officials at Vnukovo International Airport in the Russian capital of Moscow introduced a COVID-19 express testing system, whereby arriving and departing travellers can pay to receive a COVID-19 test and receive the results within an hour.
- Spanish authorities placed the municipality of Aranda de Duero under new lockdown restrictions to slow the spread of coronavirus. Residents will be prevented from leaving the area, and non-residents will be barred from entering.
- Swiss authorities reached an agreement with the American biotechnology company Moderna to secure 4.5 million doses of the company's potential COVID-19 vaccine.
- British authorities imposed several lockdown restrictions on the city of Preston after a surge in the rate of infection there; under the restrictions, people from different households will not be allowed to meet indoors or in private gardens.

8 August

- Authorities in the French capital of Paris announced that face masks will be mandatory in popular tourist destinations, including along the River Seine, the Canal Saint-Martin, the Montmartre and outdoor markets from August 10 for a month due to rising coronavirus cases in the country.
- The German Foreign Office added the Bulgarian provinces of Blagoevgrad, Dobrich, Varna and the Romanian counties of Argeș, Bihor, Buzău, Neamț, Ialomița, Mehedinți and Timiș to a list of places deemed to have unsafe levels of

coronavirus transmission, thus requiring all returning travellers to undergo a mandatory COVID-19 test.

- The Ukrainian government closed the border with the disputed territory of Crimea for three weeks to attempt to prevent the spread of coronavirus; only residents of Crimea who have Ukrainian citizenship will be permitted to enter the peninsula.
- The Australian state of Victoria has reported 466 new cases and 12 deaths.
- The Canadian province of Ontario has reported 70 new cases.
- Malaysia has reported 7 new cases, bringing the total to 9,070. 47 cases have recovered, bringing the total number of recovered to 8,775. There are 170 active cases, with two in intensive care and one of them on ventilator support. The death toll remains 125.
- New Zealand has reported no new cases, with the number of active cases remaining 23 and the total number of cases remaining 1,569 (1,219 confirmed and 350 probable cases). The number of recovered remains 1,524 and the death toll remains 22.
- Singapore has reported 132 new cases, bringing the total to 54,929.
- Ukraine has reported record-high 1,489 new daily cases as well as 27 new daily deaths, bringing the total numbers to 79,750 and 1,879 respectively; a total of 43,655 patients have recovered.
- 750,000 coronavirus test kits manufactured by Randox are being recalled due to safety concerns.

- The British Antarctic Survey announces it is scaling back its research operations because of the COVID-19 pandemic.
- The use of face coverings is extended to more indoor venues in England and Scotland.
- Schools reopened in the Gaza Strip with strict hygiene regulations in place; the Education Ministry stated that classes would be limited to four a day and schools would initially hold remedial classes only.
- Authorities in the French capital of Paris announced that face masks will be mandatory in popular tourist destinations, including along the River Seine, the Canal Saint-Martin, the Montmartre and outdoor markets from August 10 for a month due to rising coronavirus cases in the country.
- The German Foreign Office added the Bulgarian provinces of Blagoevgrad, Dobrich, Varna and the Romanian counties of Argeș, Bihor, Buzău, Neamț, Ialomița, Mehedinți and Timiș to a list of places deemed to have unsafe levels of coronavirus transmission, thus requiring all returning travellers to undergo a mandatory COVID-19 test.
- Italian Prime Minister Giuseppe Conte revealed a 25 billion euro economic stimulus package. Under the package, greater tax benefits will be granted to the poorer southern regions, cruise holidays will be resumed from August 15, monthly emergency payments to vulnerable families will be extended, and 500 million euros will be allocated to overtime payments for healthcare workers.
- The Australian state of Queensland's closure of its border with New South Wales came into force at 1 am local time. Most visitors from New South Wales will be denied entry apart from rare exceptions. Queenslanders returning to the

state will have to pay for 14 days in mandatory hotel quarantine.

- The Algerian government announced a further easing of coronavirus lockdown restrictions, with bans on non-essential travel lifted across much of the country to the end of the month, with the night-time curfew shortened. Mosques with capacities greater than 1,000 people will be permitted to reopen from August 15.

9 August

- The Australian state of Victoria has reported 394 new cases and 17 deaths. New South Wales has reported 10 new cases, bringing the total to 3,672.
- The Canadian province of Ontario has reported 79 new cases.
- Malaysia has reported 13 new cases, bringing the total to 9,083. Nine patients have been discharged, bringing the number of recovered to 8,784. There are 174 active cases while the death toll remains 125.
- New Zealand has reported no new cases, with the number of active cases remaining 23 and the total number of cases remaining 1,569 (1,219 confirmed and 350 probable cases). The number of recovered remains 1,524 and the death toll remains 22.
- Singapore has reported 175 new cases, bringing the total to 55,104.
- Ukraine has reported 1,199 new cases and 18 new deaths, bringing the total numbers to 80,949 and 1,897 respectively; a total of 43,972 patients have recovered.

- The daily figure of confirmed new COVID-19 infections exceeds 1,000 for the first time since June, rising by 1,062 to 310,825, but it is unclear whether the rise is down to a higher infection rate or a greater volume of testing.
- Sandwich chain Pret a Manger confirms it has asked thousands of members of its staff to work fewer hours as part of its plans for post-pandemic restructuring.
- British Prime Minister Boris Johnson stated that the reopening of schools in England after the summer break in September is a "moral duty" and a "national priority", due to the impact of the COVID-19 pandemic on education, and insisted that it is safe to reopen the country's schools.
- The Executive Director of Oxfam in Brazil, Katia Maia, urged international and domestic authorities to conduct an investigation into Brazil's recorded coronavirus deaths, which passed 100,000 on August 8, as well as the perceived failure of President Jair Bolsonaro and other government ministers in dealing with the pandemic.
- British Prime Minister Boris Johnson stated that the reopening of schools in England after the summer break in September is a "moral duty" and a "national priority", due to the impact of the COVID-19 pandemic on education, and insisted that it is safe to reopen the country's schools.
- The Indian Medical Association urged Prime Minister Narendra Modi to provide adequate care for healthcare workers and their families after almost 200 doctors were reported to have died from COVID-19.
- The North Korean Government delivered aid packages comprising food and medical equipment to the city of Kaesong, close to the South Korean border after a state of

emergency was imposed in July due to concerns over a possible imported case, although authorities did not confirm whether the suspected patient tested positive.

- Authorities in Malawi announced that bars and places of worship will be forced to close to slow the increasing spread of coronavirus in the country; face masks will also be mandatory in all public areas and social gatherings will be limited to ten people. The Attorney General stated that law enforcement officers will be dispatched to ensure that the public complies with the new restrictions.

10 August

- Brazil tops 3 million COVID-19 cases.
- The Canadian Province of Ontario reports 115 new COVID-19 cases.
- Malaysia has reported 11 new cases, bringing the total number to 9,094. 19 patients have been discharged, bringing the number of recovered to 8,803. The death toll remains at 125.
- New Zealand has reported no new cases. Two patients have recovered, bringing the total number of active cases to 22 and the total number of recovered to 1,526. The death toll remains 22.
- Singapore has reported 188 new cases, bringing the total to 55,292.
- Ukraine has reported 1,008 new cases and 25 new deaths, bringing the total numbers to 81,957 and 1,922 respectively; a total of 44,359 patients have recovered.
- The United States of America surpasses 5 million COVID-19 cases.

- The Director-General of the World Health Organization (WHO) pointed to 'green shoots of hope' in the pandemic while stressing two main WHO recommendations, that "leaders must step up to take action and citizens need to embrace new measures".

11 August

- The Canadian province of Ontario has reported 33 new cases.
- Malaysia has reported 9 new cases, bringing the total to 9,103. Six patients were discharged, bringing the total number of recovered to 8,809. The death toll remains at 125.
- New Zealand has reported 1 new case in managed isolation, bringing the number of active cases to 21 and the total number of cases to 1,570 (1,220 confirmed and 350 probable). The number of recovered remains 1,526 while the death toll remains 22. Later that day, four cases of community transmissions were reported, the first cases outside of a managed isolation facility for 102 days.
- Singapore has reported 61 new cases, bringing the total to 55,353.
- Ukraine has reported 1,158 new cases and 29 new deaths, bringing the total numbers to 83,115 and 1,951 respectively; a total of 44,934 patients have recovered.
- The number of global coronavirus cases has exceeded 20 million, over 12 million have recovered, and 735,000 have died.
- The International Organization for Migration and the International Chamber of Commerce released new employer guidance for measures to protect migrant workers.

- The Red Cross Society of the Democratic People's Republic of Korea deployed over 40,000 volunteers to assist North Korean urban areas in all nine of the country's provinces, including the locked-down city of Kaesong, in preventing any outbreaks of coronavirus, as well as helping with flood relief efforts.
- Disputed President of Venezuela Nicolás Maduro extended the country's state of alert by a further thirty days to attempt to slow the spread of coronavirus.
- Australian Prime Minister Scott Morrison stated that internal border closures imposed around the country were not likely to be lifted before the end of the year.
- Mayor of the Philippine capital of Manila, Isko Moreno, announced that authorities will distribute one million face masks to residents to attempt to slow the spread of coronavirus in the city; it was also revealed that the city government had allocated 200 million pesos to secure doses of potential COVID-19 vaccines.
- Office for National Statistics figures reveal that the number of people in work fell by 220,000 between April and June, the largest drop in employment in a decade. Prime Minister Boris Johnson warns there is a "long, long way to go" before the economy begins to improve.
- After the Scottish Government announces upgrades for thousands of Higher results that were marked down to take account of teachers' assessments, the National Union of Students calls for the same rules to be applied to A-Level results for the rest of the UK.
- Germany's Federal Foreign Office extended warnings advising against all non-essential travel to the Spanish

autonomous communities of Madrid and the Basque Country due to rising numbers of new daily infections, thus requiring all returning travellers to quarantine for 14 days.

- Russian President Vladimir Putin announced that a COVID-19 vaccine developed by Russian scientists at the Gamaleya Research Institute of Epidemiology and Microbiology in Moscow has received approval from the drug regulators despite clinical trials not reaching the third phase, prompting international concerns over the safety of the vaccine; authorities announced that mass vaccination could begin as early as October. The World Health Organization stated that there was 'not enough evidence' to evaluate the safety and efficacy of the vaccine, and urged the Russian government to review data from the trials to ensure the safety of patients.
- Schools in Scotland began a phased reopening after being closed since March due to the coronavirus pandemic, with the first week of schooling acting as an induction week; First Minister Nicola Sturgeon stated that the aim is to have all schools fully open by August 17.
- Authorities in Bhutan imposed the first country-wide coronavirus lockdown after a returning traveller tested positive for COVID-19. Residents were instructed to only leave their homes for strictly essential reasons, and schools and offices were ordered to close.
- New Zealand Prime Minister Jacinda Ardern has announced that Auckland will be moving into an Alert Level 3 lockdown after the discovery of 4 new cases of community transmission in that city from Wednesday afternoon to Friday midnight. Under Alert Level 3, people apart from essential workers will be encouraged to work from home while most schools, public facilities, bars, restaurants, and businesses

must close by tomorrow. The rest of the country will be moving to an Alert Level 2 lockdown from Wednesday afternoon to Friday midnight.

- Prime Minister of Papua New Guinea James Marape announced plans to ease the country's coronavirus lockdown despite surging cases; it was later revealed that the lockdown imposed on the capital of Port Moresby for the past two weeks will be lifted on August 12.
- President of the Philippines, Rodrigo Duterte, praised the efforts of the developers of Russia's approved COVID-19 vaccine and stated that the country would be willing to collaborate with Russian researchers on further trials of the vaccine.
- Health officials in the Brazilian state of Paraná revealed that negotiations were ongoing with Russian authorities to enable the production of a potential COVID-19 vaccine approved by the country's drug regulator. The governor of Paraná Ratinho Júnior will meet with the Russian Ambassador to Brazil on August 12 to discuss the proposals.
- Mexican Foreign Minister Marcelo Ebrard announced that late-stage clinical trials of three different potential COVID-19 vaccines developed by American company Johnson & Johnson and Chinese companies CanSino Biologics and Walvax Biotechnology, with the aim of eventually securing doses of the vaccines once the results of the trials are published.
- In the U.S. state of Georgia, the Cherokee County School District announced that over 800 students and over 40 staff have been advised to enter a period of quarantine due to possible exposure to COVID-19.

- Health authorities in the United States revealed that an agreement has been reached with the biotechnology company Moderna to secure 100 million doses of the company's potential COVID-19 vaccine for a cost of $1.5 billion.
- Germany's Federal Foreign Office extended warnings advising against all non-essential travel to the Spanish autonomous communities of Madrid and the Basque Country due to rising numbers of new daily infections, thus requiring all returning travellers to quarantine for 14 days.
- Russian President Vladimir Putin announced that a COVID-19 vaccine developed by Russian scientists at the Gamaleya Research Institute of Epidemiology and Microbiology in Moscow has received approval from the drug regulators despite clinical trials not reaching the third phase, prompting international concerns over the safety of the vaccine; authorities announced that mass vaccination could begin as early as October. The World Health Organization stated that there was 'not enough evidence' to evaluate the safety and efficacy of the vaccine, and urged the Russian government to review data from the trials to ensure the safety of patients.
- Schools in Scotland began a phased reopening after being closed since March due to the coronavirus pandemic, with the first week of schooling acting as an induction week; First Minister Nicola Sturgeon stated that the aim is to have all schools fully open by August 17.
- The Gaza-Egypt border temporarily reopened for limited crossings after being closed since March. A spokesperson for the Palestinian Interior Ministry announced that Palestinian citizens in possession of foreign passports and

residency permits, or people with urgent medical needs, will be permitted to leave the Gaza Strip.

12 August

- The Canadian province of Ontario has reported 95 new cases.
- Malaysia has reported 11 new cases, bringing the total to 9,114. Eight patients were discharged and there are 172 active cases. The death toll remains at 125.
- New Zealand has reported 26 active cases, with the total number of cases being 1,579 (1,225 confirmed and 354 probable). Five recoveries were reported, bringing the total number to 1,531. The death toll remains at 22.
- Singapore has reported 42 new cases, bringing the total to 55,395. In addition, 800 migrant workers have been quarantined after a new case was discovered in a cleared dormitory.
- Ukraine has reported 1,433 new cases and 19 new deaths, bringing the total numbers to 84,548 and 1,970 respectively; a total of 45,686 patients have recovered.
- Figures show the UK economy shrunk by 20.4% between April and June when compared to the first quarter of the year, making it the largest slump on record and pushing the country into recession for the first time in eleven years. Chancellor Rishi Sunak describes the situation as "unprecedented".
- The Department for Education announces that students' GCSE and A-Level results will be no lower than the results of their mock exams, with the introduction of a "triple lock" system whereby the highest grade is awarded from a choice

of mock exams, teachers' assessment or exams are taken during the autumn term.

- Following a review of the way COVID-19 deaths are recorded by Public Health England, the cumulative number for the UK is reduced by 5,377 from 46,706 to 41,329. England has previously been the only part of the UK to record a death as COVID-related no matter how long it occurred after a positive result, whereas the other constituent countries have a 28-day cut-off, which England will also now use.
- Secretary-General António Guterres briefed the UN Security Council on sustainable peace and the progress of the global ceasefire, warning that COVID-19 threatened hard-won development and peacebuilding gains and "risks exacerbating conflicts or fomenting new ones".
- Secretary-General António Guterres briefed the UN Security Council on sustainable peace and the progress of the global ceasefire, warning that COVID-19 threatened hard-won development and peacebuilding gains and "risks exacerbating conflicts or fomenting new ones".
- Authorities in the Belgian capital of Brussels announced that face masks will now be compulsory in all public places for everybody above the age of twelve, with increased police checks to ensure the public comply with the new measures.
- The German Federal Foreign Office added eleven regions of Romania, including the capital Bucharest to a list of areas deemed to have unsafe levels of coronavirus transmission, thus requiring all returning travellers to enter a 14-day quarantine. In response, German Labour Minister Hubertus Heil cancelled a planned visit later in the week to meet the

Romanian Prime Minister Ludovic Orban and several other cabinet ministers.

- Italian Minister of Health Roberto Speranza announced that travellers arriving into the country from Croatia, Greece, Malta and Spain will be required to receive a COVID-19 test following a surge in cases; Colombia was also added to a list of countries to which all travel is prohibited.
- Authorities in the Belgian capital of Brussels announced that face masks will now be compulsory in all public places for everybody above the age of twelve, with increased police checks to ensure the public comply with the new measures.
- Norwegian Prime Minister Erna Solberg announced that, from August 15, all travellers returning from Cyprus, the Faros Islands, Iceland, Malta, the Netherlands and Poland, as well as several regions of Denmark and Sweden, will be required to undergo a 10-day quarantine. Solberg also stated that Norwegian citizens should avoid non-essential international travel as much as possible.
- Authorities in Uzbekistan announced that an easing of coronavirus lockdown restrictions will take place on August 15 following declining infection rates. Under the new measures, non-essential businesses, including hotels and hair salons, will be permitted to reopen, and domestic air and rail travel will resume; people will also be allowed to leave their homes for non-essential reasons.
- Health officials in the Brazilian state of Paraná reached an agreement to produce a vaccine developed by Russian researchers and approved by the country's drug regulator, despite international concern surrounding the safety and efficacy of the vaccine.

- Peruvian President Martín Vizcarra announced that a full lockdown will be reimposed on Sundays and that family gatherings will be prohibited due to a spike in coronavirus infections.
- Hong Kong's national flag carrier Cathay Pacific reported a loss of 9.9 billion Hong Kong dollars (equivalent to almost $1.3 billion) during the first half of 2020 as a direct result of international restrictions imposed to control the coronavirus pandemic.
- In New Zealand, all rest homes went into a full lockdown in response to the discovery of four community transmissions in Auckland. In addition, it was announced that all passengers travelling to and from Auckland will be required to wear face masks, and social distancing has been reintroduced at several airports across the country.
- Jordan's Interior Ministry announced that the country's only land border crossing with Syria will be closed for a week from 13 August.
- Jordan's Interior Ministry announced that the country's only land border crossing with Syria will be closed for a week from August 13.
- The Kuwaiti Government announced that the country will move into the fourth phase of reopening after the coronavirus pandemic on August 18, with non-essential businesses including gyms and beauty salons permitted to reopen, although the night-time curfew will be maintained; sports fixtures will also be allowed to resume from August 15 without the presence of spectators.

13 August

- The Canadian province of Ontario has reported 78 new cases.
- Malaysia has reported 15 new cases, bringing the total number of positive cases to 9,129. Four cases have been discharged, bringing the total number of recovered to 8,821. There are 183 active cases, while the death toll remains 125.
- New Zealand has reported 13 new confirmed cases and 1 probable case was reported, bringing the total number to 1,589 (1,238 confirmed and 351 probable). There are 36 active cases while the number of recovered remains 1,531 and the death toll 22.
- Singapore has reported 102 new cases, bringing the total to 55,497.
- Ukraine has reported a record high of 1,592 new daily cases as well as 22 new daily deaths, bringing the total numbers to 86,140 and 1,992 respectively; a total of 46,216 patients have recovered.
- A-Level grades are published for England, Wales and Northern Ireland. School and college leaders call for an urgent review after 36% of results in England are lower than teachers predicted, while 3% are two grades lower.
- The Art Fund charity awards £630,000 to eighteen museums around the UK to support projects designed to reach the public during the pandemic. They include a pop-up museum in a shopping centre, actor guides to control social distancing and exhibit boxes that can be posted to schools.
- France, the Netherlands, Monaco, Malta, Turks and Caicos, and Aruba are added to the quarantine list, requiring

travellers arriving in the UK from these countries to quarantine for 14 days as of 4.00 am on 15 August.

- The Director-General of the World Health Organization stated that the agency's main mission was now "focused on shepherding global vaccine candidates through the necessary trials", then "guaranteeing rapid, fair and equitable access" to vaccines for every country.
- The Director-General of the World Health Organization stated that the agency's main mission was now "focused on shepherding global vaccine candidates through the necessary trials", then "guaranteeing rapid, fair and equitable access" to vaccines for every country.
- The Cook Islands has closed its air border to all travellers effective midnight local time. The order is expected to be reviewed on 17 August, prior to the next scheduled flight from Auckland on 21 August.
- President of Argentina Alberto Fernández and Mexican Foreign Minister Marcelo Ebrard announced that the two countries will produce 150 million doses of a COVID-19 vaccine being developed by British pharmaceutical company AstraZeneca to supply to all Latin American countries, with the exception of Brazil; Ebrard later revealed that the number of doses could be increased to 250 million.
- Mexican Energy Secretariat Rocío Nahle García announced that she would continue to work from home and self-isolate after testing positive for COVID-19.
- In the United States, presumptive Democratic presidential nominee Joe Biden called for state governors to impose legislation mandating the wearing of face masks in all areas

and stated that all American citizens should wear masks in outdoor areas for at least the next three months.

- The Kuwaiti Government announced that the country will move into the fourth phase of reopening after the coronavirus pandemic on August 18, with non-essential businesses including gyms and beauty salons permitted to reopen, although the night-time curfew will be maintained; sports fixtures will also be allowed to resume from August 15 without the presence of spectators.
- The Africa Centres for Disease Control and Prevention announced that seven countries - Cameroon, Liberia, Morocco, Nigeria, Sierra Leone, Zambia and Zimbabwe - will begin administering COVID-19 antibody tests to begin to understand the extent of the spread of coronavirus around the continent.

14 August

- The Canadian province of Ontario has reported 92 new cases.
- Malaysia has reported 20 new cases, bringing the total number of cases to 9,149. There are 196 active cases, with 4 in intensive care and 1 on ventilator support. Seven patients have recovered, bringing the total number of recovered to 8,828. The death toll remains at 125.
- New Zealand has reported 12 new cases and one probable new case, bringing the total number of cases to 1,602 (1,251 confirmed and 351 probable). The numbered of recovered remains 1,531 while the death toll remains at 22.
- Singapore has reported 83 new cases, bringing the total to 55,580.

- Ukraine has reported a record high of 1,732 new daily cases as well as 19 new daily deaths, bringing the total numbers to 87,872 and 2,011 respectively; a total of 46,797 patients have recovered.
- The UK government signs deals for 90 million doses of potential vaccines being developed by Belgian pharmaceutical company Janssen Pharmaceutica and the US biotech company Novavax.
- Extra ferries are laid on between France and the UK as thousands of holidaymakers race to return to the UK from France before quarantine restrictions begin.
- The UK records its highest daily rate of new COVID-19 cases since 14 June, with 1,441 new cases taking the total number to 316,367.
- The opening day of schools for the new school year in the Philippines has been pushed from 24 August to 5 October due to the response of coronavirus lockdown measures in the Greater Manila Area.
- New Zealand Prime Minister Jacinda Ardern has announced that current lockdown restrictions in New Zealand will be extended by 12 days until 11:59 pm local time on 26 August. The Auckland Region will remain on Alert Level 3 while the rest of the country will remain on Level 2 for that period. In addition, Ardern announced that the country's wage subsidy scheme would be extended to protect businesses and jobs in response to the new outbreaks.

15 August

- The Australian state of Victoria has reported 303 new cases and 4 deaths.
- The Canadian province of Ontario has reported 106 new cases.
- Malaysia has reported 26 new cases, bringing the total number of cases to 9,715. Three people have recovered, and there are 219 active cases.
- New Zealand has reported 7 new confirmed cases (all community transmissions), bringing the total number of cases to 1,609 (1,258 confirmed and 351 probable) and the number of active cases to 56. The numbered of recovered remains 1,531 while the death toll remains at 22.
- Singapore has reported 81 new cases, bringing the total to 55,661.
- Ukraine has reported a record high of 1,847 new daily cases and repeated the previous record of 33 new daily deaths, bringing the total numbers to 89,719 and 2,044 respectively; a total of 47,430 patients have recovered.
- There is confusion as the exam regulator Ofqual publishes guidelines on the criteria constituting grounds for a review of results, then withdraws the advice pending a review.
- The Local Government Association urges parents to keep up-to-date with their children's vaccinations in order to ease pressure on the NHS.
- Some restaurants and pubs report they have dropped out of the Eat Out to Help Out scheme because of "hostility towards staff".
- A UN-coordinated televised and digitally streamed concert, *Pacific Unite: Saving Lives Together*, appealed for regional

leaders and citizens of the Pacific to unite as part of the global battle against COVID-19.

16 August

- The Canadian province of Ontario has reported 81 new cases.
- Malaysia has reported 25 new cases (16 imported and 9 local transmissions), bringing the total number of infections to 9,200 cases. The country also reported 28 recoveries, bringing the total number of recovered to 8,859. There are 216 active cases and the death toll remains at 125.
- New Zealand has reported 13 new confirmed (12 community transmissions and one in managed isolation), bringing the total number of cases to 1,622 (1,271 confirmed and 351 probable) and the number of active cases to 69. There are 1,531 recoveries while the death toll remains at 22.
- Singapore has reported 86 new cases, bringing the total to 55,747.
- Ukraine has reported 1,637 new cases and 26 new deaths, bringing the total numbers to 91,356 and 2,070 respectively; a total of 47,822 patients have recovered.
- The shielding programme ends in Wales; it is the last part of the UK to end its shielding programme.
- Malaysian Director-General of Health Noor Hisham Abdullah has confirmed that the Malaysian Institute for Medical Research had detected the D614G type mutation after testing 3 cases from the Sivagangga Cluster and 1 case from the Ulu Tiram Cluster. This mutation is now the dominant form of the COVID-19 virus in the pandemic.

- New Zealand Health Minister Chris Hipkins has criticised people for using social media to spread personal attacks on the family at the centre of the recent community transmissions and conspiracy theories around COVID-19.

17 August

- The Canadian Province of Ontario has reported 99 new cases.
- Malaysia has reported 12 new cases (ten local transmissions and two imported cases), bringing the total to 9,212. Seventeen have been discharged, bringing the total number of recovered to 8,876. There are 211 active cases, while the death toll remains 125.
- New Zealand has reported 9 new confirmed cases, bringing the total number of cases to 1,631 (1,280 confirmed and 351 probable) and the number of active cases to 78. A record 26,014 tests were conducted the previous day.
- Singapore has reported 91 new cases, bringing the total to 55,838.
- Ukraine has reported 1,464 new cases and 19 new deaths, bringing the total numbers to 92,820 and 2,089 respectively; a total of 48,164 patients have recovered.
- As many as three million self-employed people whose trade has been affected by the pandemic become eligible for a second government grant worth £6,570.
- Following controversy over A-Level grades, it is confirmed that both A-Level and GCSE results in England, Wales and Northern Ireland will be based on teachers' assessments.
- A study from the Institute of Fiscal Studies says that the education gap between wealthy and poor children has

widened because of the COVID-19 pandemic, and quotes a headteacher who says it could take up to two years to get children back to their correct level of education.

- New Zealand Prime Minister Jacinda Ardern has moved the country's general election from 19 September to 17 October 2020 in response to a resurgence in community transmissions. In addition, the New Zealand Parliament's dissolution was delayed until 6 September.

18 August

- The Canadian Province of Ontario reports 125 new COVID-19 cases.
- Malaysia has reported 7 new cases, bringing the total to 9,219. 26 have been discharged, bringing the total number of recovered to 8,902. There are 192 cases and the death toll remains 125.
- New Zealand has reported 13 new confirmed community transmission cases, while 1 previous probable case was reclassified as under investigation. This brings the total number of cases to 1,643 (1,293 confirmed and 350 probable) and the number of active cases to 90. The number of recovered remained 1,531 while the death toll remains 22.
- Singapore has reported 100 new cases, bringing the total to 55,938.
- Ukraine has reported 1,616 new cases and 27 new deaths, bringing the total numbers to 94,436 and 2,116 respectively; a total of 48,925 patients have recovered.
- Education Secretary Gavin Williamson says he is "incredibly sorry" for the distress caused to students over their grades.

- The Director-General of the World Health Organization warned against "vaccine nationalism" in the COVID-19 pandemic, stating that he had written to WHO Member States, urging them to join the COVAX Global Vaccines Facility, a mechanism to guarantee fair access to effective immunization for all countries.

19 August

- The Canadian province of Ontario has reported 102 new cases.
- Malaysia has reported 16 new cases, bringing the total number to 9,235. 23 have recovered, bringing the total number of recovered to 8,925. There are 185 active cases and the death toll remains 125.
- New Zealand has reported 9 new cases, bringing the total number of cases to 1,631 (1,280 confirmed and 351 probable) and the number of active cases to 78. Five people are in hospital, an increase of two from the previous day.
- Singapore has reported 93 new cases, bringing the total to 56,031.
- Ukraine has reported record-high 1,967 new daily cases and 28 new daily deaths, bringing the total numbers to 96,403 and 2,144 respectively; a total of 49,737 patients have recovered.
- After France makes the wearing of face coverings compulsory for most workplaces, Health Secretary Matt Hancock says there are no plans to do the same in the UK.
- Pearson Education delays the release of half a million BTEC qualifications, due tomorrow, in order to regrade them.

- The UK government announces plans to expand the Office for National Statistics' Infection Survey, which tests people fortnightly for COVID-19; tests will increase from 28,000 people in England to 150,000 by October.

20 August

- The Canadian Province Of Ontario has reported 76 new cases.
- Malaysia has reported 5 cases, bringing the number of active cases to 183 and the total number to 9,240. Seven cases have recovered, bringing the total number of recovered to 8,932. The death toll remains 125.
- New Zealand has reported 5 new confirmed cases, bringing the total number of cases to 1,654 (1,304 confirmed and 350 probable) and the number of active cases to 101. Six people are in hospital, an increase of one from the previous day. The number of recovered remains 1,531 while the death toll remains at 22.
- Singapore has reported 68 new cases, bringing the total to 56,099.
- Ukraine has reported a record-high 2,134 new daily cases and a record-high 40 new daily deaths, bringing the total numbers to 98,537 and 2,184 respectively; a total of 50,441 patients have recovered.
- Portugal is added to the quarantine exemption list, while Croatia, Austria and Trinidad and Tobago are taken off it; Scotland also removes Switzerland from its own quarantine exemption list.
- The World Health Organization (WHO) and UNICEF, citing research, urged African governments to promote a safe

return of schoolchildren to classrooms while limiting spread of COVID-19.

- New Zealand Health Minister Chris Hipkins has rebuffed rumours within the Māori and Pacific Islander communities that the Ministry for Children (Oranga Tamariki) was taking away children whose relatives had tested positive for COVID-19.

21 August

- The Canadian province of Ontario has reported 131 new cases.
- Malaysia has reported 9 new cases, bringing the number of active cases to 179 and the total number of cases to 9,249. 13 have recovered, bringing the total number of recovered to 8,943. The death toll remains at 125.
- New Zealand has reported 11 new cases (9 community transmissions and two imported cases), bringing the total number of cases to 1,665 (1,315 confirmed and 350 probable). Seven new recoveries were reported, bringing the total to 1,538 and the number of active cases to 105.
- Singapore has reported 117 new cases, bringing the total to 56,216.
- Ukraine has reported 2,106 new cases and 23 new deaths, bringing the total numbers to 100,643 and 2,207 respectively; a total of 51,078 patients have recovered.
- Booking a driving test resumes in England and Wales, but the website through which bookings are made crashes due to excessive demand.
- Figures released by the Government Office for Science and the Scientific Advisory Group for Emergencies show the R

number to be between 0.9 and 1.1, up from between 0.8 and 1.0 the previous week.

- STA Travel, a firm with 50 high street outlets and specialising in trips for students and young people, becomes the latest business to cease trading because of the COVID-19 pandemic.
- Irish Agriculture Minister Dara Calleary resigned after attending a social event with the country's golf society, which may have breached Ireland's COVID-19 restrictions.
- The Food and Agriculture Organization and the World Food Programme, citing data showing that over 3 million people are facing acute food insecurity due to COVID-19 and conflict, called for urgent, sustained humanitarian action in Burkina Faso. As global cases of COVID-19 topped 22 million cases, with 780,000 deaths, and with several countries experiencing fresh COVID-19 outbreaks, the World Health Organization urged countries "to quickly identify and prevent clusters, to prevent community transmission and the possibility of new restrictions".

22 August

- The Canadian province of Ontario has reported 108 new cases.
- Malaysia has reported 8 new cases (three imported and 5 community transmissions), bringing the number of active cases to 183 and the total number to 9,257. Four patients have recovered, bringing the total number of recovered to 8,949. The death toll remains at 125.
- New Zealand has reported 6 new confirmed cases were reported, bringing the total number of cases to 1,671 (1,321 confirmed and 350 probable) and the number of active cases

to 111. The number of recovered remains 1,538, while the death toll stands at 22.

- Singapore has reported 50 new cases, bringing the total to 56,266.
- Ukraine has reported record-high 2,328 new cases and 37 new deaths, bringing the total numbers to 102,971 and 2,244 respectively; a total of 51,735 patients have recovered.
- Sir Mark Walpole, a member of the government's Scientific Advisory Group for Emergencies (SAGE), suggests that COVID-19 will be present "forever in some form or another", and not eliminated by vaccine as in the case of diseases such as smallpox.

23 August

- The Canadian province of Ontario has reported 115 new cases.
- India tops 3 million COVID-19 cases.
- Malaysia has reported 10 new cases (8 imported and 2 local transmissions), bringing the total number to 9,267. There are 183 active cases, with 9 in intensive care and two requiring ventilator assistance. 10 have recovered, bringing the total number of recovered to 8,959. The death toll remains 125.
- New Zealand has reported 3 new cases (one community transmission and two imported), bringing the total number of cases to 1,674 (1,324 confirmed and 350 probable) and the number of active cases to 114. The number of recovered remains 1,538 while the death toll stands at 22.
- Singapore has reported 87 new cases, bringing the total to 56,353.

- Ukraine has reported 1,987 new cases and 27 new deaths, bringing the total numbers to 104,958 and 2,271 respectively; a total of 52,235 patients have recovered.
- The UK's chief medical officer, Dr Chris Whitty, says that children are more likely to be harmed by not returning to school in September than by contracting COVID-19.
- The National Education Union, the UK's largest teaching union, calls for more staff, extra teaching space and greater clarity on how to deal with a spike in COVID-19 cases in order for schools to safely reopen again.

24 August

- The Canadian province of Ontario has reported 105 new cases.
- Malaysia has reported 7 new cases (5 community transmissions and two imported), bringing the total number of cases to 9,274. There are 184 active cases, with 8 in intensive care and 5 on ventilator support. Six people have recovered, bringing the total number of recovered to 8,965. The death toll remains at 125.
- New Zealand has reported 8 new confirmed cases (7 community transmissions and one imported) and 1 probable case, bringing the total number of cases to 1,683 (1,332 confirmed and 351 probable) and the number of active cases to 123. Ten people are in hospital, an increase of one from the previous day. The number of recovered remains 1,538, while the death toll remains 22.
- Singapore has reported 51 new cases, bringing the total to 56,404.

- Ukraine has reported 1,799 new cases and 22 new deaths, bringing the total numbers to 106,754 and 2,293 respectively; a total of 52,524 patients have recovered.
- As schools in Northern Ireland return for the autumn term, Prime Minister Boris Johnson releases a message to parents telling them it is "vitally important" children go back to school, with the life chances of a generation at stake.
- A University of Bristol study finds that young teenagers aged 13 and 14 experienced less anxiety during lockdown than they did in October 2019.
- Tesco announces the creation of 16,000 new jobs following an "exceptional growth" in its online business during the lockdown.
- UN Secretary-General António Guterres launched his latest policy brief on tourism, calling for the vital global tourism sector to be rebuilt in a "safe, equitable and climate-friendly way". The WHO urged greater investment in the global COVID-19 vaccine facility, the COVAX Global Vaccines Facility, which 172 countries are now participating in and which aims to deliver two billion doses in 2021. UN Special Rapporteurs and Independent Experts on human rights have raised the alarm over the “grave and unnecessary” risks of catching COVID-19 faced by imprisoned human rights defenders facing lengthy pre-trial detention in Egypt.
- The WHO announced only a slim possibility of COVID-19 reinfection, citing documented cases of 1 in over 23 million.
- New Zealand Prime Minister Jacinda Ardern has announced that Auckland would remain under a Level 3 lockdown until 11:59 pm on 30 August, when the city and the Auckland Region would move to a Level 2 lockdown. The rest of New

Zealand will remain on a Level 2 lockdown until 6 September. From 30 August onwards, it will be compulsory for all people using public transportation to wear face masks.

25 August

- The Canadian province of Ontario has reported 100 new cases.
- Malaysia has reported 11 new cases, bringing the total number of cases to 9,285. There are 189 active cases, with 8 admitted into intensive care and 6 of them requiring ventilator support. Six have recovered, bringing the total number of recovered to 8,971.
- New Zealand has reported 7 new community confirmed cases, bringing the total number of cases to 1,690 (1,339 confirmed and 351 probable) and the number of active cases to 129. One new recovery was reported, bringing the total number of recoveries to 1,539.
- Singapore has reported 31 new cases, bringing the total to 56,435.
- Ukraine has reported 1,658 new cases and 25 new deaths, bringing the total numbers to 108,415 and 2,318 respectively; a total of 52,870 patients have recovered.
- Scientists at the University of Nottingham have identified a 75-year-old woman from Nottinghamshire whom they believe to be the first person to catch COVID-19 through transmission within the UK; she tested positive on 21 February.
- Virgin Atlantic receives £1.2bn backing from its creditors to keep operating for at least another 18 months and save 6,500 jobs.

- Figures produced by the Treasury show that the Eat Out to Help Out scheme has been used 64 million times during the first three weeks of August.

26 August

- The Canadian Province Of Ontario has reported 88 new cases.
- Malaysia has reported 6 new cases (5 community transmissions and 1 imported), bringing the total to 9,291. There are 188 active cases, with 9 in intensive care and 6 on ventilator support. Seven have recovered, bringing the total number of recovered to 8,978. The death toll remains at 125
- New Zealand has reported 5 new cases (three community transmissions and two imported) bringing the total number of cases to 1,695 (1,344 confirmed and 351 probable) and the number of active cases to 134. The number of recovered remains 1,539 while the death toll stands at 22.
- Singapore has reported 60 new cases, bringing the total to 56,495.
- Ukraine has reported 1,670 new cases and 36 new deaths, bringing the total numbers to 110,085 and 2,354 respectively; a total of 53,454 patients have recovered.
- A BBC survey of the UK's largest employers identifies fifty that say they have no immediate plans to return all their staff to the office.
- Research carried out by the Defence Science and Technology Laboratory suggests that insect repellent that contains Citriodiol could be used to kill a strain of coronavirus that triggers COVID-19.

- Restaurant chains, including Prezzo, Harvester and Pizza Pilgrims, announce plans to extend the Eat Out to Help Out scheme into September due to its success, saying they will fund it themselves once the government-backed scheme ends.
- Prime Minister Boris Johnson blames a "mutant algorithm" for the exam grades chaos.
- Jonathan Slater, the chief civil servant at the Department of Education, is dismissed from his position over the exams controversy.
- New Zealand Health Minister Chris Hipkins has announced that it will be compulsory for all public transport providers including buses, trains, ferries, ride-share vehicles and train operators to provide Covid Tracer QR codes from 11:59 pm on 3 September.

27 August

- The Canadian province of Ontario has reported 118 new cases.
- Malaysia has reported 5 new cases, bringing the total to 9,296. 16 have recovered, bringing the total number of recovered to 8,994. There are 177 cases, 8 in intensive care and 6 needing respiratory assistance. The death toll remains at 125.
- New Zealand has reported 7 new confirmed cases (6 from the community and 1 imported), bringing the total number of cases to 1,702 (1,351 confirmed and 351 probable). 15 new recoveries were reported, bringing the total to 1,554 and the number of active cases to 126. The death toll remains 22.

- Singapore has reported 77 new cases, bringing the total to 56,572.
- Ukraine has reported 1,974 new cases and record-high 49 new daily deaths, bringing the total numbers to 112,059 and 2,403 respectively; a total of 54,217 patients have recovered.
- The number of new daily COVID cases rises by 1,522, the highest number since mid-June.
- The delayed Liberal Democrats leadership election sees Sir Ed Davey elected to lead the party.
- Switzerland, Jamaica and the Czech Republic are removed from the quarantine exemption list effective from 4 am on 29 August, while Cuba is added to it as a destination from where travellers will not need to quarantine.
- Sandwich chain Pret a Manger announces the loss of 3,000 jobs in a bid to save the business.
- The Royal Shakespeare Company cancels its theatre productions until 2021 because of the pandemic.
- A YouGov poll suggests support for the full-time reopening of schools in England and Wales has risen from 57% to 65% over a three-week period.
- The WHO has announced the setting up of an independent expert Review Committee to examine aspects of the international treaty that governs preparedness and response to health emergencies. UNAIDS has warned in a new report, Rights in a pandemic – Lockdowns, rights and lessons from HIV in the early response to COVID-19, that some of the world's most marginalized communities have experienced violence and other rights abuses during the COVID-19 pandemic.

- New Zealand Health Minister Chris Hipkins has announced that it would be compulsory for everyone over the age of 12 to wear face masks on trains and planes from 31 August. However, exemptions will be granted for health, disability, and practicality reasons. Violators face a NZ$300 infringe notice or a fine of NZ$1,000.

28 August

- The Canadian province of Ontario has reported 122 new cases.
- Malaysia has reported 10 new cases, bringing the total number to 9,306. There are 151 active cases, with 8 in intensive care and 6 on ventilator support. 36 have recovered, bringing the total number of recovered to 9,030. The death toll remains 125.
- New Zealand has reported 12 new confirmed cases (5 from the community and 7 imported), bringing the total number of cases to 1,714 (1,363 confirmed and 351 probable). Seven new recoveries were reported, bringing the total to 1,561 and the number of active cases to 130.
- Singapore has reported 94 new cases, bringing the total to 56,666.
- Ukraine has reported record-high 2,438 new cases and 48 new daily deaths, bringing the total numbers to 114,497 and 2,451 respectively; a total of 55,083 patients have recovered.
- The UK government announces the launch of another drive to encourage people to return to their workplaces, starting in the first week of September.

- The BBC Two's current affairs programme *Newsnight* is given access to a SAGE document that suggests a "reasonable worst-case scenario" may be to expect 85,000 COVID deaths over the coming winter.
- Malaysian Prime Minister Muhyiddin Yassin has announced that the country's Recovery Movement Control Order restrictions would be extended until 31 December 2020.

29 August

- The Canadian Province of Ontario report 148 new COVID-19 cases.
- Malaysia has reported 11 new cases, bringing the total number of cases to 9,317. Eight people have recovered, bringing the total number of recovered to 9,038. There are 154 active cases, with 8 in intensive care and 6 on ventilator support. The death toll remains at 125.
- New Zealand has reported 13 new confirmed cases (11 community transmissions and 2 imported), bringing the total number of cases to 1,727 (1,376 confirmed and 351 probable). 7 new recoveries were reported, bringing the total to 1,568 and the number of active cases to 137. The death toll remains at 22.
- Singapore has reported 51 new cases, bringing the total to 56,717.
- Ukraine has reported record-high 2,481 new cases and 41 new daily deaths, bringing the total numbers to 116,978 and 2,492 respectively; a total of 56,138 patients have recovered.

- The first football match with spectators takes place in Brighton, with 2,500 people allowed in to watch a pre-season friendly between Chelsea and Brighton.
- Women's football makes a return for the first time since lockdown, with a Community Shield match between Chelsea and Manchester City, the first Women's Community Shield to be held since 2008.

30 August

- The Canadian province of Ontario has reported 112 new cases.
- Malaysia has reported 17 new cases, bringing the total number to 9,334. 1 death was reported, bringing the death toll to 126. Ten people were discharged, bringing the total number of recovered to 9,048. There are 160 active cases, with 7 in intensive care and 5 of these on ventilator support.
- New Zealand has reported two new confirmed cases (both community transmissions), bringing the total number of cases to 1,729 (1,378 confirmed and 351 probable). Two new recoveries were reported, bringing the total to 1,570. The number of active cases remains at 137 while the death toll remains 22.
- Singapore has reported 54 new cases, bringing the total to 56,771.
- Ukraine has reported 2,096 new cases and 35 new daily deaths, bringing the total numbers to 119,074 and 2,527 respectively; a total of 56,734 patients have recovered.
- A total of 25 million cases, over 16 million recoveries, and 850,000 deaths have been reported globally.

- As a million students prepare to go to university, the Universities and Colleges Union urges universities in the UK to delay face-to-face lectures until after Christmas amid concerns students could spark a second wave of the COVID pandemic.
- Emily Eavis, the co-organiser of the Glastonbury Festival, says the organisers aim to stage Glastonbury 2021 in June 2021 as usual.
- A further 1,715 cases of COVID-19 are reported, bringing the total so far to 334,467, and representing the largest daily increase since mid-may. A single death brings the total number of fatalities to 41,499.
- Guernsey's Vale Earth Fair is held as usual at Vale Castle, attended by 3,500 people but with its lineup of performers being entirely from Guernsey.
- New Zealand Prime Minister Jacinda Ardern confirmed that the country's largest city Auckland would enter into "Alert Level 2.5" from 11:59 pm on Sunday night while the rest of the country would remain on Level 2. Under Level 2.5, all social gatherings will be limited to ten people; masks will be mandatory for all Aucklanders using public transportation, and aged care facilities will be operating under strict conditions.

31 August

- The Canadian province of Ontario has reported 114 new cases.
- Malaysia has reported 6 new cases, bringing the total number of cases to 9,340. Six have recovered, bringing the total number of recovered to 9,054. 1 new death was

reported, bringing the death toll to 127. There are 159 active cases, with 6 in intensive care and 4 on ventilator support.

- New Zealand has reported 9 new cases, bringing the total number of cases to 1,738 (1,387 confirmed and 351 probable). 15 new recoveries were also reported, bringing the total to 1,585. There are 131 cases with 11 people in the hospital. The death toll remains at 22.
- Singapore has reported 41 new cases, bringing the total to 56,812.
- Ukraine has reported 2,141 new cases and 30 new daily deaths, bringing the total numbers to 121,215 and 2,557 respectively; a total of 57,114 patients have recovered.
- The Eat Out to Help Out scheme comes to an end. Over 100 million meals were eaten under the scheme, at a cost to the government of about £522 million. A University of Warwick study later concluded that some areas with high scheme uptake had increased new infections after about a week and that 8% to 17% of new infection clusters could be linked to the scheme.
- Airline operator Tui launches an investigation after sixteen passengers on a flight from Zante to Cardiff subsequently test positive for COVID-19, amid claims safety measures were ignored on the flight.
- The Reading and Leeds Festivals, cancelled in 2020 because of the COVID-19 pandemic, announce plans for their 2021 festivals from 27 to 29 August 2021.

The WHO Director-General warned that kickstarting economies without a COVID-19 plan was a 'a recipe for disaster', while advising on the measures that individuals, communities and government, communities could take to ensure safety. Addressing a virtual town hall with young women from NGOs, part of the annual session of the Commission on the Status of Women, coordinated by UN Women, the UN Secretary-General stated that the COVID-19 pandemic had reversed decades of fragile progress on gender equality and women's rights.

References

Responses to the COVID-19 pandemic in August 2020 (2021) Wikipedia. Available at: https://en.wikipedia.org/wiki/Responses_to_the_COVID-19_pandemic_in_August_2020 (Accessed: 2 May 2021).

Responses to the COVID-19 pandemic in July 2020 (2021) Wikipedia. Available at: https://en.wikipedia.org/wiki/Responses_to_the_COVID-19_pandemic_in_July_2020 (Accessed: 22 May 2021).

Responses to the COVID-19 pandemic in June 2020 (2021) Wikipedia. Available at: https://en.wikipedia.org/wiki/Responses_to_the_COVID-19_pandemic_in_June_2020 (Accessed: 2 May 2021).

Responses to the COVID-19 pandemic in May 2020 (2021) Wikipedia. Available at: https://en.wikipedia.org/wiki/Responses_to_the_COVID-19_pandemic_in_May_2020 (Accessed: 2 May 2021).

Timeline of the COVID-19 pandemic (2021) Wikipedia. Available at: https://en.wikipedia.org/wiki/Timeline_of_the_COVID-19_pandemic (Accessed: 20 April 2021).

Timeline of the COVID-19 pandemic in Afghanistan (2021) Wikipedia. Available at: https://en.wikipedia.org/wiki/Timeline_of_the_COVID-19_pandemic_in_Afghanistan (Accessed: 20 April 2021).

Timeline of the COVID-19 pandemic in Argentina (2021) Wikipedia. Available at:

https://en.wikipedia.org/wiki/Timeline_of_the_COVID-19_pandemic_in_Argentina (Accessed: 20 April 2021).

Timeline of the COVID-19 pandemic in August 2020 (2021) Wikipedia. Available at: https://en.wikipedia.org/wiki/Timeline_of_the_COVID-19_pandemic_in_August_2020 (Accessed: 20 April 2021).

Timeline of the COVID-19 pandemic in Australia (2021) Wikipedia. Available at: https://en.wikipedia.org/wiki/Timeline_of_the_COVID-19_pandemic_in_Australia (Accessed: 20 April 2021).

Timeline of the COVID-19 pandemic in Bangladesh (2021) Wikipedia. Available at: https://en.wikipedia.org/wiki/Timeline_of_the_COVID-19_pandemic_in_Bangladesh (Accessed: 20 April 2021).

Timeline of the COVID-19 pandemic in Belarus (2021) Wikipedia. Available at: https://en.wikipedia.org/wiki/Timeline_of_the_COVID-19_pandemic_in_Belarus (Accessed: 20 April 2021).

Timeline of the COVID-19 pandemic in Brazil (2021) Wikipedia. Available at: https://en.wikipedia.org/wiki/Timeline_of_the_COVID-19_pandemic_in_Brazil (Accessed: 7 May 2021).

Timeline of the COVID-19 pandemic in Canada (2021) Wikipedia. Available at: https://en.wikipedia.org/wiki/Timeline_of_the_COVID-19_pandemic_in_Canada (Accessed: 7 May 2021).

Timeline of the COVID-19 pandemic in Croatia (2021) Wikipedia. Available at:

https://en.wikipedia.org/wiki/Timeline_of_the_COVID-19_pandemic_in_Croatia (Accessed: 7 May 2021).

Timeline of the COVID-19 pandemic in England (January–June 2020) (2021) Wikipedia. Available at: https://en.wikipedia.org/wiki/Timeline_of_the_COVID-19_pandemic_in_England_(January–June_2020) (Accessed: 10 March 2021).

Timeline of the COVID-19 pandemic in England (July–December 2020) (2021) Wikipedia. Available at: https://en.wikipedia.org/wiki/Timeline_of_the_COVID-19_pandemic_in_England_(July–December_2020) (Accessed: 20 May 2021).

Timeline of the COVID-19 pandemic in Fiji (2021) Wikipedia. Available at: https://en.wikipedia.org/wiki/Timeline_of_the_COVID-19_pandemic_in_Fiji (Accessed: 10 March 2021).

Timeline of the COVID-19 pandemic in Ghana (2021) Wikipedia. Available at: https://en.wikipedia.org/wiki/Timeline_of_the_COVID-19_pandemic_in_Ghana (Accessed: 10 March 2021).

Timeline of the COVID-19 pandemic in India (2021) Wikipedia. Available at: https://en.wikipedia.org/wiki/Timeline_of_the_COVID-19_pandemic_in_India (Accessed: 5 June 2021).

Timeline of the COVID-19 pandemic in Indonesia (2021) Wikipedia. Available at: https://en.wikipedia.org/wiki/Timeline_of_the_COVID-19_pandemic_in_Indonesia (Accessed: 5 June 2021).

Timeline of the COVID-19 pandemic in Japan (2021) Wikipedia. Available at: https://en.wikipedia.org/wiki/Timeline_of_the_COVID-19_pandemic_in_Japan (Accessed: 22 February 2021).

Timeline of the COVID-19 pandemic in July 2020 (2021) Wikipedia. Available at: https://en.wikipedia.org/wiki/Timeline_of_the_COVID-19_pandemic_in_July_2020 (Accessed: 22 February 2021).

Timeline of the COVID-19 pandemic in June 2020 (2021) Wikipedia. Available at: https://en.wikipedia.org/wiki/Timeline_of_the_COVID-19_pandemic_in_June_2020 (Accessed: 15 January 2021).

Timeline of the COVID-19 pandemic in Malaysia (2021) Wikipedia. Available at: https://en.wikipedia.org/wiki/Timeline_of_the_COVID-19_pandemic_in_Malaysia (Accessed: 15 January 2021).

Timeline of the COVID-19 pandemic in May 2020 (2021) Wikipedia. Available at: https://en.wikipedia.org/wiki/Timeline_of_the_COVID-19_pandemic_in_May_2020 (Accessed: 22 February 2021).

Timeline of the COVID-19 pandemic in Mexico (2021) Wikipedia. Available at: https://en.wikipedia.org/wiki/Timeline_of_the_COVID-19_pandemic_in_Mexico (Accessed: 18 April 2021).

Timeline of the COVID-19 pandemic in Nepal (2021) Wikipedia. Available at: https://en.wikipedia.org/wiki/Timeline_of_the_COVID-19_pandemic_in_Nepal (Accessed: 22 February 2021).

Timeline of the COVID-19 pandemic in New Zealand (2021) Wikipedia. Available at: https://en.wikipedia.org/wiki/Timeline_of_the_COVID-19_pandemic_in_New_Zealand (Accessed: 23 March 2021).

Timeline of the COVID-19 pandemic in Nigeria (2021) Wikipedia. Available at: https://en.wikipedia.org/wiki/Timeline_of_the_COVID-19_pandemic_in_Nigeria (Accessed: 20 May 2021).

Timeline of the COVID-19 pandemic in Pakistan (2021) Wikipedia. Available at: https://en.wikipedia.org/wiki/Timeline_of_the_COVID-19_pandemic_in_Pakistan (Accessed: 10 January 2021).

Timeline of the COVID-19 pandemic in Romania (2021) Wikipedia. Available at: https://en.wikipedia.org/wiki/Timeline_of_the_COVID-19_pandemic_in_Romania (Accessed: 10 February 2021).

Timeline of the COVID-19 pandemic in Russia (2021) Wikipedia. Available at: https://en.wikipedia.org/wiki/Timeline_of_the_COVID-19_pandemic_in_Russia (Accessed: 23 February 2021).

Timeline of the COVID-19 pandemic in Singapore (2021) Wikipedia. Available at: https://en.wikipedia.org/wiki/Timeline_of_the_COVID-19_pandemic_in_Singapore (Accessed: 23 February 2021).

Timeline of the COVID-19 pandemic in Spain (2021) Wikipedia. Available at: https://en.wikipedia.org/wiki/Timeline_of_the_COVID-19_pandemic_in_Spain (Accessed: 23 February 2021).

Timeline of the COVID-19 pandemic in Sweden (2021) Wikipedia. Available at: https://en.wikipedia.org/wiki/Timeline_of_the_COVID-19_pandemic_in_Sweden (Accessed: 16 May 2021).

Timeline of the COVID-19 pandemic in Thailand (2021) Wikipedia. Available at: https://en.wikipedia.org/wiki/Timeline_of_the_COVID-19_pandemic_in_Thailand (Accessed: 16 May 2021).

Timeline of the COVID-19 pandemic in the Philippines (2021) Wikipedia. Available at: https://en.wikipedia.org/wiki/Timeline_of_the_COVID-19_pandemic_in_the_Philippines (Accessed: 20 May 2021).

Timeline of the COVID-19 pandemic in the Republic of Ireland (2021) Wikipedia. Available at: https://en.wikipedia.org/wiki/Timeline_of_the_COVID-19_pandemic_in_the_Republic_of_Ireland (Accessed: 23 February 2021).

Timeline of the COVID-19 pandemic in the United Kingdom (January–June 2020) (2021) Wikipedia. Available at: https://en.wikipedia.org/wiki/Timeline_of_the_COVID-19_pandemic_in_the_United_Kingdom_(January–June_2020) (Accessed: 23 March 2021).

Timeline of the COVID-19 pandemic in the United Kingdom (July–December 2020) (2021) Wikipedia. Available at: https://en.wikipedia.org/wiki/Timeline_of_the_COVID-19_pandemic_in_the_United_Kingdom_(July–December_2020) (Accessed: 23 February 2021).

Timeline of the COVID-19 pandemic in the United States (2020) (2021) Wikipedia. Available at: https://en.wikipedia.org/wiki/Timeline_of_the_COVID-19_pandemic_in_the_United_States_(2020) (Accessed: 10 march 2021).

Timeline of the COVID-19 pandemic in Trinidad and Tobago (2021) Wikipedia. Available at: https://en.wikipedia.org/wiki/Timeline_of_the_COVID-19_pandemic_in_Trinidad_and_Tobago (Accessed: 19 May 2021).

Timeline of the COVID-19 pandemic in Turkey (2021) Wikipedia. Available at: https://en.wikipedia.org/wiki/Timeline_of_the_COVID-19_pandemic_in_Turkey (Accessed: 19 May 2021).

Timeline of the COVID-19 pandemic in Uruguay (2021) Wikipedia. Available at: https://en.wikipedia.org/wiki/Timeline_of_the_COVID-19_pandemic_in_Uruguay (Accessed: 23 February 2021).

Timeline of the COVID-19 pandemic in Vietnam (2021) Wikipedia. Available at: https://en.wikipedia.org/wiki/Timeline_of_the_COVID-19_pandemic_in_Vietnam (Accessed: 15 January 2021).

World Health Organization's response to the COVID-19 pandemic (2021) Wikipedia. Available at: https://en.wikipedia.org/wiki/World_Health_Organization%27s_response_to_the_COVID-19_pandemic (Accessed: 10 January 2021).

https://www.telegraph.co.uk/global-health/science-and-disease/wuhan-officials-identified-huanan-market-pandemic-risk-least/

CPSIA information can be obtained
at www.ICGtesting.com
Printed in the USA
LVHW050138160222
711264LV00009B/404

9 781915 206886